10 *Vital*

TO LIVING AN EXTR/

BE YOU

THE STRATEGIC GUIDE TO THE
Ultimate Natural You

REG LENNEY
The Multi-Award-Winning Vital Coach

Praise for Reg Lenney

"Thanks Reggie for helping me to return to beauty and full power in the physical... It's a miracle... You will ALWAYS have my heartfelt gratitude for believing in my full power, beauty and strength and insisting I live it. Like no other you are supporting me to rediscover all of this in the physical after a prolonged terminal lung disease which had left me bedridden on oxygen for 24 hours... where I was given 12 hours to live 3 times! I feel a new passion igniting in us both to truly assist others – watch out world!!!! Smiles... two givers, two highest achievers, finally learning to receive from each other... I believe in happy endings now."

—**Dr Susie Anthony**, after being told by 'specialists' 7 years ago that she would not make it to her next birthday

♦♦♦

"I believe! I have never experienced such complete relief and immediate results; you are a true healer..."

—**Halle Berry**

♦♦♦

"I met Reg four years ago, hoping to improve my physical fitness and nutritional health. I received so much more than that. Reg delivered a full spiritual, emotional and physical reboot that allowed me to get into a heightened state of awareness about all of the conditions of my life. Solutions to lifelong problems began to flow shortly thereafter.

I learned how to live with passion, in the flow, and I had the physical energy to do it. Reg is that rare person, a teacher and a learner. He never stops seeking to improve his own ability to deliver peak performance for his clients. His methods come from both timeless tradition and cutting edge research. I am very grateful."

– **Tim Corcoran**

"Thanks mate. You are a true healer and the best of the best!"

—**Hugh Jackman**

✦✦✦

"I will make this short and simple; I was diagnosed with lung cancer which was at 'an advanced stage'.

My doctor told me it was very aggressive and was spreading through-out my body, I could last as long as 6 months. The suggestion was to do chemo therapy, which was not a "cure" but would give me an extra few months to live. I have seen many friends go through the chemo therapy and decided to not put my body or my family through that.

I had been told about you by some friends and after much encouragement from my family I decided to give you a try. The first 3 months were a big life change along with a learning experience about myself; this experience could never be explained in words, it must be experienced.

I have now been following your program and enjoying your services for over 2 years now and to my delight, my families delight and my doctors amazement, the cancer has completely cleared up. I feel better then I have felt in years and am living a fuller life then I ever have. I recommend you and your health program to any one living with pain or disease or any one living half of a life. You have not only helped me to "cure" my body, you have helped me to move out of my shell, move out of my routine, move beyond my limits and be a better person then I ever thought I could be.

Thank you for giving my life back to me and my family."

—**Gerard B.**

✦✦✦

"After my very first session I slept 12 hours..and woke up today, hive less, FYI.. for the first time in months. THANK YOU. I am so excited about the rest of my program and look forward to learning and growing with you. Blessings."

—**Erin French**

acknowledgments

This book is dedicated first and foremost to my two beautiful children, Amanda, and Brittany. I love you and I have always wanted you in my life, and I will always love you and wish for you to be in my future. You are forever on my mind and in my heart. I wish you were in my life now and I look forward to the day your hearts and minds are open to the truth and reality of why you have been separated from your family who loves you more than words could ever express. We all miss you and are here when you are ready.

Secondly, to all those who I have had the privilege to work with, learn from, and grow with me over the past 32 years—and all those I look forward to working with in the future. Your passion and strength have encouraged me to know more and be better, and your success fuels me with passion and persistence. I am very proud of you all!

My mother, 'mommee,' the reason I am and have become. My rock, my teacher, my support, my truest and best friend, the one I have always looked up to, who has always inspired me, who has always held me accountable to being the best version of me possible, and who has allowed me to fall far below so as to guide me through the lesson. I love you! Thank you for being you, and for sharing you with me!

Last, but certainly not least—Yolanda, my angel, my love, my partner, the one who is consistently encouraging me, supporting me to grow, expand and become a better version of myself every day. I love you, I cherish you, I admire your strengths, and I am grateful for all you are and all you share with me. Your daily love, laughter and support is my magic. I am grateful to have you by my side, joining me in my journey and allowing me to join you in yours. Your amazing children Clara and Carlos are consistently helping me to see life in exciting new ways. I am more aware of how looking at life through the eyes of a child can keep my mind clear of stress, fear, worries and limitations. Every minute of every day is exciting, full of possibilities, and a clean slate where anything can happen. Children don't automatically think the worst when presented with new situation, idea's, opportunities and choices, and this is an exciting and powerful way to live life, and what BE YOU! is all about. Sharing my time with Clara and Carlos have reinforced the importance of choosing to be happier, healthier, more positive and the best version of ourselves throughout all aspects of our life, no matter what happened in the past, what mistakes we make or how long it takes to become the individual we really want to be. Understanding the power of a positive mind, together with the realisation that every minute of every day we have choices, which either take us towards the life we love, or away from it, have encouraged me to never stop asking myself "What do you want to be when you grow up?" at any age.

contents

foreword

Be You is an introduction to a new way of thinking; an integration of East and West, ancient wisdom and modern medicine, and the outcome of choice. Reg's background, interests, and life passion combine into an opportunity for every reader to learn through a combination of science and wisdom, while introducing an intuitive way of thinking about your health.

Who am I and why am I introducing you to 'Be You'?

My name is Dr. Kareem Samhouri, although most people know me by 'Kareem'. You see, I travel the world spreading the voice of personalized health and epigenetics. My companies and I reach over 1 million people on a daily basis through DrKareem.com, and I sit on the boards for many leading health companies across the world. Simply put, Reg and I have a common interest in ending chronic pain & disease worldwide, while helping you reach your true health capacity.

By focusing on yourself first, you set an example the world can follow to feel better.

As you read 'Be You', you may sense a bit of dissatisfaction surrounding traditional medicine, but please make no mistake about it: Reg is a huge proponent of Western Medicine, when done correctly; it's illogical traditional medicine he refutes. In fact, Reg lost his father to medicine gone wrong; his father's doctor didn't understand the value of lifestyle choices and how they affect survival rate with a terminal diagnosis.

Logically, you may understand that your attitude, environment, diet, thoughts, feelings, and support system affect your ability to heal or feel better, even when you have a common cold, let alone if you have a terminal illness. We all 'get it'; now is the time to take 'intuitive knowledge' and integrate it into the medical model. And fortunately for us, Reg is leading the way.

You'll begin to understand mind patterns trigger emotions that release chemicals in your body, thereby exciting your nervous system and heightening your attention and likelihood to lash out, respond, or run away. You'll see that 'everything' in your life is a sign of health, and every moment of your day is an opportunity to choose you.

In fact, this is an emerging area of science called 'Epigenetics'. For many years, the conversation has been about genetics, or your genes. suggesting that your genes determine your health, or your potential health. Well, that's not entirely true.

You see, your genes + your environment = you, or your phenotype.

This means the decisions you make on an every day basis—such as where you live, what you do, who you talk to, when and what you eat, how and how much you move, what you're thinking about and feeling, and whether or not you're living with purpose—all affect your health. Each one of these aspects of 'health redefined' constitute 'epigenetic influences' on your genes. And every 2-3 minutes, your genes are turning on or off.

Effectively, every 2-3 minutes you have an opportunity to affect your health in a positive way and express 'only' your very best genes. When you take responsibility for conversations, feelings, thoughts, and choices, great health becomes the default.

And it becomes obvious you are unique. Through discovering your uniqueness, you will be able to reach your health potential.

In 'Be You', Reg goes over 10 keys to optimize health that will forever simplify your approach. No matter how healthy—or unhealthy—you ever get, you can rely on these ten keys to help you; this form of wisdom only comes through education, trial & error, time, and the sheer volume of clients Reg has helped.

Reg has learned through personal experience that the quality of your life experience is directly proportional to the state of your health. When relationships are great, you're having fun, you're loving life—and you are actively taking care of your body and mind—life is incredible. Likewise, it's important to realize that toxic conversations and relationships are affecting you on a physiological level; and that your physiology is affecting your relationships in a toxic way. Fortunately, breaking the cycle is easy: pay attention to how you feel and the choices you make throughout the day.

As soon as you see that choosing 'you' is both about survival *and* quality of life—and that it's ok for everyone else to choose *themselves* too—you'll feel a lot lighter. No more expectations on others to manage, and you no longer have to prioritize other people's needs and desires over your own health and prosperity.

'Be You' presents a very complete—and simple—approach to health. And, it's fully engaging and interesting to read. You'll love the adventure Reg takes you on while you learn to discover the 'health code' for your body and mind.

Congratulations, Reg, on an incredible book. And thank you so much for sharing your wisdom with the world. This is truly a life's work, and it's extremely gracious of you to share your health message.

Dr. Kareem F. Samhouri
DrKareem.com

We are all human beings who are dealing with similar core issues that affect how our bodies and minds work. This is why health professionals can help, because when we learn about the human body, the mind, and the soul, when we are ready, we can understand how it feels to be human.

We discover eventually that there is no "one-size-fits-all" when it comes to health, happiness, fulfillment, or success. We see this often in emergency situations, and I should know, having been professionally involved in this field for more than 10 years.

We are all unique and different, so you simply can't do what everyone else is doing and expect it to work the same way for you. Unfortunately, this is what the biomedical model of Western medicine has to offer. So then, we must let go of the belief in one single solution, a solution that is valid for all.

Reg and I go back many years. We both wanted to understand more, to do our best at helping, caring, and healing. I am a holistic medicine clinician, and after 40 plus years of practice, I can say that Reg is one of few that I met, who has dedicated his life to his clients.

When he writes that we all need to look honestly into our own lives, and if we discover that we are not living the life we really are meant to live, the life we could live, the happiness we all long for, what does it mean?

It means we need to change.

Which change you may ask?

Your partner, your job, your government? Well, it's not reasonable to expect that to change any time soon.

Yes, you already guessed it: it's ourselves we need to work on. Difficult to admit? Perhaps, yes. Necessary? I am afraid so. But fear not, because change is not as painful as it looks. Under the right guidance it becomes easier with time, with repetition and training. As they evolve, your beliefs as they evolve will make change possible by adapting and supporting your efforts.

Before you realize, your life will have changed. You will have reclaimed who you really are.

I admit that for a very long time, I was bitterly complaining about my own life. I did what my duty dictated and that allowed me the secondary benefits of not having to make the changes. Yes, it was painful. I won't deny it. But man, what a relief when I finally admitted that I had it all in me: ideas, solutions, power, and most importantly, the core desires for my life.

All that I needed to do was take a closer look at the beliefs that weren't working for me in all the different areas of my life.

You too should also examine the limiting beliefs, those that don't inspire you to be better. Beliefs truly are the core to the entire Natural You approach. You have the power and the right to make the changes that will support you. You have the right to be exactly who you want to be.

Dr. Dominique Dock

preface

For over 32 years, I have dedicated my life to helping people understand the importance of the choices we make every day and how they impact our overall health. I believe in commitment. Committing to small, easy steps all day every day and consistent advancement towards your goal rather than setting unattainable and unsustainable goals for yourself. When you set goals that are too difficult to maintain long-term, you are setting yourself up to fail. This cycle of big goal setting without a system to support you in maintaining your results will lead to repeated failure. This can leave a person feeling stuck, overwhelmed, and insecure.

I hope to encourage and educate everyone to understand how the small changes we make, in service to the longer-term goals we wish to reach, create the biggest impact in our lives and help us move forward. Most importantly, I invite people to notice the choices they make that will potentially destroy any chance of long term health, success, and happiness.

My intention is to help you to stop "trying" this or that and to get clear about what is right for you. One-size-fits-all approaches don't work because they're not what's best for *you*. The best systems and strategies are those that will encourage and support you to maintain your excellence, your growth, and your passion. When you incorporate these into your daily life and every choice you make, they will ultimately ensure your success.

You can choose to "live with it," "die from it," or "change it," but you do have a choice in your health and the life you are living. I'm going to educate you on alternatives to conventional health, fitness, and medicine that make sense and really work, as proven to me by thousands of clients over the years. It is never too late to turn your health and your life around if you just open your mind and give it a chance.

The definition of insanity is doing the same things over and over while expecting different results. So, let's do things a little differently.

Change doesn't take place in a day, but every day you can enjoy improvement and victory as you grow closer to your goals.

Finally, a disclaimer: I work with severe cases of bodily injuries and health issues. I trained for 7 years in India, 3.5 years in eastern Asia and over 14 years in Canada and the USA, consistently upgrading my skills and knowledge to stay ahead of this changing world and how our bodies react to it, focusing on the energy, power, and communication through the body. I specialize in muscle and energy balancing and the communication from the brain through the body. My clients have had fantastic success with what seemed to be impossible situations.

However, **this book is not intended as a substitute for the medical advice of physicians**. The reader should regularly consult a physician in matters relating to his/her health and particularly with respect to any symptoms that may require diagnosis or medical attention. What I teach in this book should be followed in conjunction with your doctor's orders.

Your power and Ultimate Health come from clarity, knowledge, and the understanding of how to keep your body and mind functioning to the best of their ability. All the opinions expressed in this book are those of the author and are meant to be just those—opinions. Ultimately, my mission for this book is to make you aware of what may be affecting your health, and to show you alternative ways to take control of it, rather than learning to "live with it" or "die from it." It's up to you to decide what to do with your newfound knowledge. The Author and Publisher assume NO LIABILITY for any loss or damage suffered because of the use, misuse, or reliance on the information provided in this book.

Thank you for your time, and I look forward to taking this journey with you.

—Reg

"

Be yourself, but always
your better self.

—KARL G. MAESER

introduction

Everything changes, and everything affects everything...or does it?

Who are you?

Are you someone who has created a life where you:

- are dealing with your life,

- are suffering from your life,

- are living with unfulfilled dreams,

- are living with failed relationships,

- have been passed by on that promotion,

- are unrecognized talent,

- have every reason to feel happy and fulfilled... but you don't feel it,

- are stuck in a rut of living a life you wish would or could change,

- are forced into a life change by a tragedy, a change you never saw coming or that just finally happened,

- feel like change is happening all around you, but you don't know how to maintain your mental and physical performance so you can keep up, keep doing what you love in the lifestyle you have worked so hard for, or still wish to achieve,

- are held back by limiting beliefs; you're still trying to live the life you were told to live, in the way you were told to live it, but it just doesn't feel right,

- have worked hard for many years to achieve your goal, only to realize it's not what you want, or it's not what you thought it would be,

- spent most of your life focused on your work, duties, and dreams, only to see that you are now truly alone, unhealthy, and unhappy,

- have just kept your head down and my mouth shut...but you just can't do it anymore, but you don't know where to go next,

- have seen so many "specialists," read so much information, heard so many different ideas and how-to's, and now have a whole lot of incomplete and bad information,

- keep trying to create the life you really want, in the body you really want, with the energy, passion, and fulfillment you really want, only to experience more failure, frustration and disappointment,

- have "specialists" telling you this is the way it is...you have to learn to live with it, or you're going to die from it, or

- have spent countless amounts of money, hired many "specialists" or "coaches," taken all the courses, gone to all the events, bought all the t-shirts...but you just can't make it the way you want it?

Is there really a way to live the life you want and love the life you live?

Can you really eliminate chronic aches, pains, ailments, and disease, or do you just keep living with them?

Whether you're dealing with life issues, health issues, career issues, relationship issues or old age and the changing world around you, there is a simple way to achieve your goals and find your own path to happiness and fulfillment, without spending tons of money, stressing yourself out, or diving deep into all the 'hokey pokey holistic and new-age stuff.'

Change is inevitable. Over time, your body, your beliefs, your wants, and your needs have changed, and they will continue to change, as will your perception, attitude, and general emotional state—and not necessarily for the better. But, you do have a choice as to how you change. You truly can be in control of your health and all aspects of your life, and it doesn't need to be hard.

Ask yourself, "Am I still thinking in the same ways that I was conditioned to as a child?

"Has my health or the reality of the life I have created to this point suddenly caught up with me?

"Have I ever really stopped to ask myself, 'Is what I'm doing with my life and the way I am doing it worth it? Is it what I really want to be doing, with the people I'm doing it with, for the rest of my life? And, do I really want it anyway?'"

| Change is inevitable.

Is it really true that getting the body and/or the life you want needs to be hard work, scary, time-consuming, expensive or nearly impossible to achieve?

What about the constant strain on your relationship(s)? You're finding it difficult to love yourself and keep the romance alive with others. Are you living with the wrong person or people? Or, are you finding it hard to meet someone new because you feel unattractive physically, you just don't see the point, you haven't got the energy, and your self-confidence is non-existent these days? This feelings and beliefs only add to your stress and makes you feel even grizzlier.

Does any of this sound at all familiar?

What Does This Mean for You?

You don't have to be stuck, unfulfilled, frustrated, sluggish, ill, overweight, suffering from an ailment or disease or feeling like an old, grouchy grizzly bear, whether you are 17, 25, 32, 45, 59, 75 or even older.

You have so much more control over the quality of your life and your destiny than you have been brought up and conditioned to believe, and I can show you how. You are not destined to simply go wherever the universe takes you. You don't have to believe what you have heard or been taught. You don't have to do things that make you unhappy simply because you think you're supposed to do them. You do have a choice and you can make a change, and change can often happen a lot faster than you believe, even sometimes immediately.

Whether your goals are to get to the next level of performance and power, hold onto your success, maintain your lifestyle, hold off old age, recover from injury, eliminate ailments and disease, lose weight, change your body shape, improve your strength, get healthy, stay healthy pre- or post-pregnancy, cope with life's stresses, totally change your life, create the life you want from where you are now, or just generally feel more fulfilled, energized, and alive, or something else completely, what you learn in this book will help you understand and experience how tiny little steps and tiny little changes can make a massive impact on your life right now. And, you'll learn how you can maintain those changes long term.

> ## You have so much more control over the quality of your life and your destiny than you have been brought up and conditioned to believe, and I can show you how.

Learning how to take control, make the changes, and meet your goals just takes a little bit of education, awareness, and honesty.

In this book I will guide you through the simple steps, or as I like call them, the "Vital Keys" to achieving and maintaining health, happiness, and fulfillment." These are the keys that I have learned throughout more than three decades of courses, training, education, and real-life experiences, both on my own journey as well as working with the incredible people I have had the opportunity to share my time with and learn from. These keys are what I've taught to hundreds and hundreds of clients to help them live and maintain their best possible lives. I will share with you how consistently making simple little choices will put you firmly in control of all areas of your life. You will ultimately learn how to become a better, healthier, happier, and more fulfilled natural you. This book is your opportunity to share in some of my real-life experiences that will show you how you too can achieve exceptionally high levels of mental and physical performance, while consistently achieving the life you truly want. Let me show you how.

> I often wonder why more people don't focus on attaining a consistent record of great health. Instead, they focus on maintaining, surviving, and coping with ailment, pain, and disease.

First, let's talk about health.

How often do you hear about an organization raising money to 'cure' an ailment or disease? Rarely, if at all. In fact, in some parts of the world, it is illegal to even mention the word "cure." In advertising and promotion of "health issues," practitioners are not permitted to say or present anything using the word "cure." What a strange world we live in. Have you ever asked yourself why that is?

Over the last year alone, there have been reports of over 80 doctors, scientists, and specialists mysteriously disappearing or dying shortly after releasing details of a "cure." Many doctors I work with have stated that when they were in school, "you were at no time allowed to talk about a cure." These doctors are trained in allopathic medicine, which is the treatment of disease by conventional means.[1] Allopathic medicine often results in the prescription of drugs that have effects that are directly opposite to the symptoms you're experiencing.

Our medical system is not designed to get people healthy, it's designed to maintain and/or create ailment and illness to keep the cash flowing in. Don't believe me? Research it for yourself with an open mind and see just how much money is being created by ill-health and how much money would be lost with a cure.

---

[1] Allopathy [Def. 1]. (nd.). In Merriam Webster Online, Retrieved July 11, 2017, from http://www.merriam-webster.com/medical/allopathy.

LET ME BE CLEAR: I am not anti-medicine. I believe that Western medicine has a time and a place, and this book certainly should not take the place of any medical advice. What I do advocate is doing your own research and not blindly following advice or instructions if you're not seeing the results you want. Educate yourself, and don't be afraid to ask for a second opinion. Be true to the Natural You.

I often wonder why more people don't focus on attaining a consistent record of great health. Instead, they focus on maintaining, surviving, and coping with ailment, pain, and disease. Why are all the scientifically-altered, pre-packaged, pre-made, genetically-modified, easy-to-access, cost-effective convenience foods and products filling the shelves and restaurants when they have been proven to create so many mental and health issues in our world today? Why are we not only making it easier to make ourselves sick, but also consistently choosing to support the industries creating it?

Our medical system is not designed to get people healthy, it's designed to maintain and/ or create ailment and illness to keep the cash flowing in.

Generally, we believe that the government and organizations like the FDA are looking out for our best interests and doing all they can to keep us safe and healthy. But if this is the case, then why is there little or no research into natural cures and proven alternative options? Why is it that anyone making a claim about anything natural is mocked and ostracized? Why are all the natural products being outlawed? And why is sugar permitted and purposely put in everything, under countless names and titles, including "healthy" foods, even though it has been proven to cause and worsen serious health issues? Medical science has demonstrated that sugar is up to eight times more addictive than heroin and cocaine.[2] If the government, the FDA, and big business were really concerned with people's health, rather than how much money they can make, wouldn't it be easier to get nutritious natural foods and products that promote peak performance, and at a lower cost?

The problem as I see it is that we have all these fundraising events going on to raise money for "research." But, it seems like the only things they are researching are more drugs, treatments, and ways to maintain our health problems instead of researching preventative medicine and ancient healing modalities that have worked for thousands of years.

Think of what would happen to the "cancer industry" if a cure were released. Can you imagine the amount of lost money, the number of lost jobs, or how many big businesses would go bankrupt? For decades, doctors and scientists have proven they can cure cancer, yet these people disappear or are ostracized and their work is destroyed. If big business really wanted to find a cure, why wouldn't these people be hailed as heroes, or at least have their work studied endlessly to improve it, and bring it to those in need, rather than having that research stopped entirely?

This is what the medical system is all about—learning to "live with it" rather than helping people move from the ill state to the healthy state. If I ended up with cancer or any other ailment or issue, I wouldn't want to learn to live with it. I would want to learn how to be free from it. Just as important, I would want to know why I got there in the first place.

Why are we not only making it easier to make ourselves sick, but also consistently choosing to support the industries creating it?

It's the same with a physical injury or a mental illness. There are a lot of massage therapists, chiropractors, doctors, psychiatrists, counselors, and other specialists who keep busy because they have many

---

[2] Sullum, J. (2013, October 17). Research Shows Cocaine and Heroin Are Less Addictive Than Oreos. Retrieved August 15, 2017 from https://www.forbes.com/sites/jacobsullum/2013/10/16/research-shows-cocaine-and-heroin-are-less-addictive-than-oreos/#54626c402427.

clients coming back to them. Week after week, month after month, year after year, they 'help' their clients dealing with identical issues, just trying to maintain their state and manage their pain. In fact, often these "specialists" are praised for being very successful in their business and being great at what they do.

Let's analyze this for a minute. I was once asked to share an office with a very well-known and respected chiropractor. I thought it would be a great idea to team up with another specialist who wanted to help people maintain high levels of health. To my great surprise, after two weeks I was asked to move out of his office. Why? Because he told me I was "fixing people too fast." What!? I had never heard of such a thing. I thought that was exactly what we were meant to do. However, he told me that for every client I "fixed," he needed to spend money on advertising to replace them.

The reality is, part of the training these "specialists" receive teaches them how to create a base of regular clients coming in repeatedly. A successful "specialist" is often looked at as someone who has a schedule that is so full of regular clients that they can't take any new ones. In fact, the busier a "specialist" is with regular clients, the more the public believes these "specialists" are great. The "best" doctors are so busy, it's almost impossible to get an appointment, unless you know someone or have the right titles. Is this in the best interest of the patient, or the "specialist's" bank account?

> If you're in the health or improvement business, you should be in the change, healing, or "cure" business.

Personally, I see that as a colossal failure. If you're in the health or improvement business, you should be in the change, healing, or "cure" business. That means you shouldn't have "regular clients" dealing with the same issues for long periods of time. I don't want my clients coming to see me for months or years, dealing with the same issues. I want to help them change and heal quickly, enjoy and experience high levels of mental and physical performance, so they can get going on creating the rest of their life in the way they want to be living it. That's exactly what I'm going to try to teach you to do in the remainder of this book.

Throughout this book I would like to share some information that could change your life . . . and that could save you a lot of time, confusion, frustration, heartache, and money, and ensure you are in control of your life, your health, happiness, and your future long term.

The information I will share with you can help you to increase your brand value, help you to advance your business or career, and earn more money in less time. This book will help you to spend time with your family and loved ones, doing the things that you enjoy doing. It will help you increase your natural energy levels, improve your immune system, and help to repair your body and mind so they work more efficiently. With this book, you'll even learn how to take your fitness and fat loss to the next level. This book will give you the control over your life and health now and in the future. It's your guide to ultimate happiness, success, and health.

The 10 Keys to Ultimate

1. BELIEFS & CHOICES

Beliefs are the most important area of your life and/or business. What you believe directly affects your perception of the world, your core values, and your life choices. The power to change your life is in your beliefs. Beliefs play a huge role in the choices you will make in your everyday life. But, when you make the right choices that support the life you want to live, you'll find that you become the best version of yourself naturally.

2. ASSESSMENT

Once you consider your beliefs and choices, you must assess all of the areas of your life. Are they helping you get closer to living the life you love and loving the life you live, or are they keeping you from it?

3. BODY WISDOM & THERAPY

What do your body and mind need, and what are the best strategies and techniques to enhance, repair, restore, rejuvenate, and empower them?

4. LIFESTYLE

What kind of life are you living now? What kind of life do you *really* want? The choices you make every moment of every day either take you towards the goals you want or take you away from them. The people you spend the most time with, the things that you focus on, and your beliefs are what create the lifestyle you live. Look at your life. Are you happy? Do you feel successful? Do you love waking up every morning and coming home every night?

5. ENVIRONMENT

Your environment can make you stressed out, sick, and fat, and it has a dramatic impact on your happiness, health, and success—in your business, your family, and your overall life. The environments in which you spend the most time have a major effect on whether or not you achieve the results you want in every aspect of your life. Reflecting on the environments you grew up in, have a career in, and live in will open the door to understanding the changes you can make to live an extraordinary life that you love and are passionate about.

Happiness, Success, and Health

6. NUTRITION

It's no secret that eating well will support your overall health, but it can also drastically affect your happiness, stress levels, success, and a lot more. Fuel your body and mind for the results you want to see in your life.

7. FITNESS

You need to do the right exercise, at the right times, in the right ways. Exercise means different things to different people. We all have different ways we enjoy working out and keeping fit to feel great. Whether it is working out hard in a gym or at home, or if you prefer to find alternative methods of toning your body and keeping your muscles loose, strong, healthy, and balanced, find what works for you and what's fun for you. Then, keep doing it.

8. RELATIONSHIPS

The people you spend your time with have an enormous effect on your ability to live a truly extraordinary life. Take the time to assess your relationships, and to examine your beliefs surrounding those relationships.

9. DETOXING

You should systematically detox your body in the way it needs to support you in achieving the best version of you. Cleansing/detoxing based on a latest fad or single-function cleansing will not serve your body or mind appropriately, and often can create more problems and issues. You need to holistically cleanse your body using tried and true methods like the ones outlined in this book.

10. SUPPORT SYSTEM

How many times have you embarked on a journey to transform something in your life? Have you ever bought a self-help book, taken courses, or gone to an energetic event where you were told all the things you could be and do if you would just take the right steps? If so, you've probably found the changes were difficult, if not impossible, to maintain. Why did you fail? It's probably because you didn't have the right support.

The Best Version of the Natural You

"

Every little action
creates an effect: We
are all interconnected.

—YEHUDA BERG

Your Body Is Holistic—
So Is Your Life!

Your life and your health are your choice. To really understand your health, how to be healthy, why you get sick, and how to stay healthy, you must look at your body as the sum of all parts. Conventional medicine is often lacking when it comes to examining the emotional, environmental, and spiritual elements of our life that can harm or help us in our health quest. Once you set forth to have a balanced life in all areas, not only to follow the conventional path towards health (if you choose), but also to focus on a healthy mindset and environment, you will begin to see the changes and impacts you have been seeking in your life. This chapter covers my journey to discover the power of a holistic approach, my unique approach to helping you find and maintain health, happiness, and success in all areas of your life holistically (which I call the Natural You approach), and the natural and holistic connection between the mind, body, and environment.

Living a Life You Love, Loving the Life You Live

I'm sick and tired of seeing people sick and tired. I've seen so many clients who have fallen from high levels of success, or they never even achieve that success. I see people suffering and becoming overweight, depressed, and downright miserable. Often there is absolutely no reason why they should be suffering. If they make the right choices and choose the right help, guidance, and information, they can absolutely get better. Later in the book, I'll share with you some incredible life transformation stories and experiences.

| Your body doesn't exist in isolation.

My approach is holistic. It's not necessarily a spiritual approach; rather, it is a whole person approach. Everything you believe in and surround yourself with, everything you eat, how and when and why you eat, how you feel about things, how you react to things, the choices you make, the way you deal with stress and how you view the world all have a positive and negative influence on your life and your goals. That may seem overwhelming, but it's also a good thing! It means that ultimately you are in control of your health, and you have the power to change your health and your life if you're not happy with it.

Let's begin by looking at why your body needs a natural approach to living and an integrated approach to health, happiness, and success. You'll learn why the holistic approach is the most powerful way to maintain and improve your health. We will explore why you are forever connected to the planet's natural systems. And, we'll discuss why you must tend to your own natural systems for them to maintain optimal functionality.

Your body doesn't exist in isolation. Your surroundings, your mind, your beliefs, your emotions, and the foods and substances that you choose to put *into* and *onto* your body all affect your body's different systems. The limbic system, the nervous system, the immune system, and the cardiovascular system all work in conjunction and synchronous relation with one another, and they're all affected by the health and lifestyle choices you make. They may be distinct systems, but whether they're working well and working efficiently individually affects how they work as a whole, which affects your overall health.

You are also a result of your parents, their beliefs, your upbringing, and your surroundings. Where you have come from and by those who you spend time with have formed your beliefs, habits, and lifestyle. When you begin to understand how those beliefs affect your overall health, and how your thoughts and emotions can either make you sicker or make you healthier, you begin to truly understand the power your parents and family really have over you. Your childhood affects your adulthood and the way you feel and deal with everything in your world.

To make changes to your life, to become happier and healthier, you need to look at everything about you and where you came from. If you are not happy with "you" or you want to take "you" to new levels of health and performance, then you need to create new spaces, new habits, and make new choices to take you there. This book will guide you through the process of discovering what has been holding you back, and how you can move past all of that to create a new, better you.

If you're not getting the results you want—physically, mentally, emotionally or financially, in all areas of your life—it's because you have not been told the whole truth, or what you have been doing isn't working for you. The first step is to be *aware* of how your environment and mind have a huge impact on your health. You must understand what truly affects your health so you can understand what you need to change to become your best self.

Why Do We Become Ill?

It's become painfully obvious to me that despite growing awareness, there is something clearly missing from conventional medicine. The world still seems to be clueless about the bigger picture of why we get sick and how to eliminate it. Despite centuries of medical research, we're still getting sick, and in large numbers. The conventional approach isn't working, but most people just don't realize it.

Popular media opinion on health, whether from an allopathic perspective or a natural, more alternative perspective, sadly still focuses almost exclusively on the physical body and the symptoms. Whenever the media does discuss emotional, mental, or spiritual components, these issues are often skirted over and generally countermanded with a scientific or medical opinion—which usually softens, if not negates, the former.

We are told to follow guidelines to live a healthy life, such as taking our vitamins, getting plenty of rest and exercise, eating a balanced diet and avoiding stress. In fact, you've probably followed these recommendations yourself, but you still find that you're not quite where you want to be. So why doesn't this approach work? We'll cover that in detail, but first, let me tell you a little about my own journey and perspective.

My Father's Illness

It all started with my father being diagnosed with brain cancer, which happened before I was born. The first 15 years of my life, I knew he had this condition and I watched him go through our medical system that either cut the top of his head off or drugged him up so much that he just wasn't himself or who he wanted to be.

My mother was very much into what we'd call today "alternative care" and "natural healing." She believed that a happy, healthy, clean, and well-balanced life, body, and diet, along with the right supplements and plenty of mental and physical exercise, were the best way to create a very strong, healthy life and body. She believed in the power of a true holistic approach.

My father's mother was different. She followed the traditional belief that the doctors knew best and you listen to what they say no matter what. She strongly believed you should only do what the doctors tell you to do. My grandmother referred to anything outside conventional Western medicine as "hokey pokey witchcraft stuff."

> My father's battle with cancer is what sparked my interest in science, medicine, traditional and alternative care and what could be the core of it all.

I saw this battle going on between two modes of thinking about health. I noticed that when my father was doing what the doctors were saying, he was either in bed or he was drugged up on the couch or he was on his hands and knees, hammering his head against the floor because his head was hurting so much. Conventional medicine told us this was "good." However, when he was doing the "hokey pokey witchcraft stuff," his hair grew back, he acted normal, he returned to work, and most important to me at the time, he was more of a father.

Watching this as a child, made me interested in how the body works and what makes us healthy or unhealthy, what makes us well or unwell. I wondered if there might be something to this "hokey pokey witchcraft stuff" after all. I remember being six years old and rubbing my dad's head, putting my hands on him and him saying that I made him feel better by massaging him. It made me think, "That's kind of odd. How does that happen?"

Some years later, he went to Mexico, when my mother heard from many different sources that they had a "cure for cancer." For over a half-century, patients have flocked to clinics in Mexico for treatments that are generally shunned, prohibited, or regarded as outright quackery in the United States and Canada. In the 70's when my Dad started going there, countless people from all around the world were going home much better than they had arrived, many claimed they had returned from Mexico "cured," and doctors saw the unbelievable, positive results.

When my dad went, his doctors took him off his myriad of pharmaceuticals and put him on this brown tonic with a couple of little natural pills. Surprisingly to everyone, he did feel better. Not only did he *feel* better, but his hair grew back, he lost a ton of weight, and he returned to work. He felt that he had beaten cancer. Tests were coming back with positive results and all seemed to be on the right track.

His return to health lasted for quite a while, but then my grandmother and her doctor thought his new treatment regimen was just masking the real problem and he needed to go back on his course of pharmaceuticals and chemotherapy. The constant fear created by my grandmother and her medical team of "specialists," the bouncing between what my mom wanted him to do and what his mom wanted him to do, and my father not being true to himself and living the life *he* really wanted to live, were more than my father could handle. The battle within his environment pushed my father to move back in with his mother. He was removed from our family home, away from my mother's "bad influence," and he began listening to what the doctors were telling him to do. This is where he spent the last two years of his life.

My mother had managed to keep him alive through 15 years of the worst part of his cancer and numerous operations, drug therapy, and other medical interventions. Her "alternative approach" of continuously detoxing and cleansing his body, feeding him clean, nourishing foods, providing natural supplements, and helping him live a healthy natural lifestyle gave him a real quality of life. It took less than two years of full-on conventional care before he was gone. I was fifteen. He was forty-three. I just turned 50 last December.

My father's battle with cancer is what sparked my interest in science, medicine, traditional and alternative care and what could be the core of it all. It also opened my eyes to the importance of looking at all aspects of a person's life and why we get sick in the first place, rather than just looking at what we end up dealing with. In short, it's what's inspired me to look at health holistically.

But what happened with many of those clinics in Mexico since those early days? The fact is that the powers of control fought back, claiming these clinics had been carrying out 'unproven treatments' and did not follow 'proper procedures.' Countless clinics closed down, endless individuals who were doing all they could to help clients with every possible option available were ostracized, arrested, forced out of business, and in many cases either died under mysterious circumstances or disappeared.

Living through my father's disease and seeing the effects of its natural and 'alternative' treatment motivated my curiosity for life, health, and understanding the choices we make every day. It inspired me to pursue becoming a medical doctor. I knew I wanted to help people, and being a medical doctor seemed like the right choice. At the time, I didn't know there were "natural doctors" or anything like that. I simply saw the conventional path, and I chose to begin to follow it.

In medical school you would always find me asking questions like: What about nutrition? What about detoxing the body? What about alkaline balance? What about simply exercising and sleeping well? What about changing your mental attitude? What about lifestyle choices and being true to yourself? What about the environment? What about the products we have in our homes and put on our bodies? I had so many questions, but I didn't receive many answers.

Instead of getting answers or an opening for discussion, I would only get people mad at me all the time. It was as if we weren't allowed to ask those types of questions. All you could discuss was what drugs to prescribe and what the conventional treatment plan would be. If I talked about anything else, I would get into trouble. I thought that was very odd and confusing. Now as an adult and now that I am more aware, I am even more confused as to why some doctors and modern medical practices mock these types of questions. Why do adults believe blindly in the medical business, and why is anyone outside of it crazy?

You see, because of my mom, I knew that the answers to my questions contributed to a person's wellbeing. And, I understood that if any of them were off balance for long periods of time, then dis-ease would arise in the body. Imbalance is the cause of ailments and illnesses, failures in relationships, and unsuccessful and unfulfilling careers. These different, seemingly common-sense things were important to me, and I wanted to make a difference in people's lives, happiness, health, and success.

Is There a Natural Cure for Disease?

As a compassionate healthcare professional, I am constantly overwhelmed by the suffering that I see daily and the "no cure" messages that are forced on us constantly. As a therapist, I am frustrated with the "there's a pill for everything" approach, along with all the false information and bad advice. As a counselor and coach, I am committed to providing accurate, understandable information without the hype.

I'm troubled by the alarming health trends of our day and age. Did you know the number of people with diabetes has risen from 108 million in 1980 to 422 million in 2014?[1] All kinds of diseases and chronic conditions have been on the rise over the past few decades, and the medical establishment hasn't provided many answers. Take, for example, a news article from August of 2017 that's headlined, for example, "Colon cancer deaths rise among younger adults, and no one knows why."[2] No one knows why?!?

What's changed in the past few decades? Over the past 20 years, kids have grown up on GMOs, and processed and fast foods. Soft drinks and sugary treats are constantly filling their bellies. Kids are being given pharmaceuticals for every little ailment, not to mention all the vaccines forced on them. Why is there a lack of fresh fruits and vegetables in their diets? Kids are stuck in front of the TV, computer, or tablet, and get driven everywhere, so they are experiencing very little physical movement for endless hours. What is that lack of movement doing to their lives?

How is it possible, with the amount of money and effort put into medical science and research, that humans are now facing all these drastic health issues in wealthy and developed countries? Why is it

---

[1] World Health Organization (2017, July). Diabetes. Retrieved from http://www.who.int/ mediacentre/factsheets/fs312/en/.

[2] Howard, J. (2017, August 9). *Colon cancer deaths rise among younger adults, and no one knows why.* Retrieved from http://www.cnn.com/2017/08/08/health/colon-cancer-rectal-cancer-deaths-study/index.html

that "common" diseases are on the rise in wealthy countries but in the countries where incomes are very low, their disease rates are very low? And, what can we learn from those countries with low disease rates to improve our own health?

> ## Did you know the number of people with diabetes has risen from 108 million in 1980 to 422 million in 2014?

Many people believe there are natural cures for disease and doctors and specialists have been making "cure" claims for years. The problem is the lack of evidence and research about natural cures. Unfortunately, the specialists, doctors and scientists around the world claiming to have the cures seem to disappear, die mysteriously, or end up in jail and labeled as crazy. The last few years alone, over 80 medical and scientific specialists who claimed to find a 'cure' have died or disappeared under very strange circumstances. Don't believe me? Do your own real research and see what you find. We are living in a world where illness, disease, pain, and suffering are on the rise, and we are left with nothing but questions and confusion.

It's obvious natural cures for disease are subject to some debate. The laws created and governed by big business are designed to support the bottom line of the medical industry. From insurance companies to hospitals to pharmaceutical companies, the system is designed to make them money. In the past 20 years, the pharmaceutical and health industries have spent over $3.5 *billion* lobbying the US government.[3] There is nothing in these statutes that encourage the doctors to get you well. How would they make money if you were healthy?

It's important to note that nothing you read here is meant to take the place of your doctor's advice. You should never discontinue a prescribed treatment without first consulting your doctor. I work very closely with my clients' doctors. In fact, I insist my clients have full scans and tests before they start working with me. I do it so the

---

[3] Center for Responsive Politics. (2017, October 21). Lobbying Top Spenders. Retrieved from https://www.opensecrets.org/lobby/top.php

doctors are aware of what we are doing. The tests and documentation are also great for showing the results and changes. However, I strongly believe there are strategies, techniques, herbs, botanicals, minerals, foods, common vitamins, and environments that help the body naturally control and heal itself. I have personally witnessed complete and full reversal of many ailments and illnesses, such as high blood pressure, diabetes, cancer, Alzheimer's, AIDS, asthma, psoriasis, ADHD, and many other "incurable" ailments and illnesses.

Curing Chronic Diseases Holistically

It's relatively easy to believe that a holistic approach can help someone who's overtired or who suffers from seasonal allergies. But what about patients who have been suffering from ill health for years or even decades? What if it was possible to reverse your ailments and disease? I will go over many such ways that it's possible to do so in this book. I invite you to explore and practice the suggestions in this book for six months, and notice how your body reacts and your life improves to this natural test. You will be your own proof that my system works.

Opponents of natural cures for chronic illnesses and diseases believe that manufacturers and authors target people suffering from those ailments, offering hope where there is none, and sometimes causing the delay of conventional or "proven" treatments. They believe that these snake oil salesmen are just out to make money selling a product that at best won't relieve their symptoms. Some proponents of natural cures claim that the federal government, pharmaceutical companies, and even the medical associations suppress information about natural remedies.

How does conventional medicine deal with a patient who's not well? Doctors typically begin by getting them on some regular routine of pills and gently suggesting weight loss, healthy diet, and physical activity. But, when a person is plagued with fatigue and feels depressed, they may not be able to follow those suggestions. Or, they may try following their doctor's orders, but they don't see any symptom relief.

What's missing in the doctors' treatment regimens that's keeping their patients from seeing results? Doctors commonly overlook factors such as their environments, lifestyle choices, bad relationships, environmental toxins including terrible air and water quality, missing vitamins and minerals, poor nutrition, and a lack of movement. Most traditional doctors almost always overlook these factors, and they dramatically downplay their importance. Three decades of experience tells me those doctors are wrong.

> My clients have had fantastic results in reversing and eliminating the symptoms of chronic conditions like diabetes because of the unique, natural lifestyle that I live by.

Doctors and nutritionists quote guidelines for "adequate" nutrition all the time, and major health organizations believe that malnutrition is rare in developed countries. Excellent, natural, unprocessed, nutritious foods, on the other hand, seems to prevent chronic diseases. And, they provide the energy and mental clarity that people need to make the choice to change their lifestyles. There are many documented cases[4] of people who have lived years beyond their medical doctor's expectations by using alternative treatment plans, changing their lifestyles, and increasing the intake of specific nutrients that remedy the condition from which they suffered.[5]

My clients have had fantastic results in reversing and eliminating the symptoms of chronic conditions like diabetes because of the unique, natural lifestyle that I live by. I believe that everything we do affects our ability to be and maintain the best natural version of ourselves. To "cure" ailments, you must deal with the whole person and what they are currently experiencing in all areas of their life, not focus only on the symptoms of an illness. To cure chronic illness, you need to work at every level, starting from belief systems to environment and relationships to supplements and nutrition. That's why my approach is so different—and why it's so effective.

---

[4] Smith, C. (2014, August 5). The Trevor Smith Story: How He Beat Bladder Cancer Naturally with Cannabis Oil. Retrieved from https://www.cureyourowncancer.org/trevor-smiths-story-how-he-beat-bladder-cancer-naturally-with-cannabis-oil.html.

[5] Axe, J. & Zielinski, E. (2017, July 31). "10 Natural Cancer Treatments I Hidden Cures." Retrieved from https://draxe.com/10-natural-cancer-treatments-hidden-cures/.

The best natural version of you is the result of an empowering and unique lifestyle. It's not only about getting a massage, exercising, or eating right. It is a combination of things that are 'right' for your mind, your body, and your heart's greatest desires. Share your time with the people, places, and things that make you feel alive, happy, and successful. You will begin to understand that the lifestyle I promote is an extraordinary lifestyle that is unique to every individual. What works for one person does not necessarily work for another. Each person is an individual and each case needs individual attention and diagnoses. But, that's also the power of this lifestyle, and that's why it actually *works*.

"Natural" Supplements Aren't Always What They Say They Are

But, a bottle of a "natural" supplement isn't always your direct ticket to health. Please read the label carefully. Health products are also very big business and you need to educate yourself before throwing your money down the toilet of "healthy" alternatives. For example, there are precise nutrients that should be present in products advertised as natural cures for type 1 diabetes, but they are not always included in supplements for diabetics. There are also specific herbal extracts and other supplements that, according to scientific studies, control blood sugar levels and prevent complications that can accompany diabetes.

Do your research and educate yourself about the supplements you're taking. Make sure you're actually getting what the bottle says is in your supplement. Always follow the manufacturer's instructions, but at the same time, do your own research so that you truly understand how much of something you should be taking in order to achieve the results you want and are paying for. If you are taking prescription medications, you should also make sure to check with your pharmacist or supplement manufacturer concerning possible interactions, and get very clear about what you are willingly putting into your body.

The Interconnected Systems

Your thoughts affect your feelings, as does your attitude. How well you maintain your various bodily systems through your choices of physical activity, nutrition, and lifestyle affects your thoughts, emotions, and attitude. Likewise, your mental state has an enormous effect on your body and how it functions. Ultimately, these elements and systems work together to take you where you will end up in life and the body in which you experience it. Together they take you not only to your destinations, but also to your destiny.

Consider people who suffer from Seasonal Affective Disorder (SAD). They tend to become fatigued or even depressed when the days become shorter and nights longer. Their bodies, minds, attitudes, and emotions are more sensitive, which means they are more affected by the conditions of light and dark. Their environment affects their mood and feelings, which then in turn affect their entire bodies.

The concept that our physical and mental health varies with the seasons and sunlight goes back centuries. *The Yellow Emperor's Classic of Medicine,* a philosophy treatise on health and disease that's estimated to have been written around 300 B.C.E., describes how the seasons affect all living things and recommends that during winter one should "retire early and get up with the sunrise. Desires and mental activity should be kept quiet and subdued, as if keeping a happy secret." In his *Treatise on Insanity,* published in 1806, the French physician Philippe Pinel noted a mental deterioration in some of his psychiatric patients "when the cold weather of December and January set in."

Most psychiatrists regard SAD as being a subclass of generalized depression, or in a smaller proportion of cases, bipolar disorder. Studies have been conducted around the world to understand the positive effect that light therapy can have. Research and testing is well-established in Sweden but they have concluded that "no satisfactory results have come from the controlled studies which have been published on the subject." They said the value of therapy with a light box for SAD "can be neither confirmed nor dismissed," which, while inconclusive, was interpreted by some as "light therapy has no effect."

The reality? Many of my clients who had been experiencing extreme cases of SAD in the past are now experiencing the seasonal change very differently. What did we do? Simply stated, we adjusted their attitude. Take cold weather as an example. I come from Canada originally. I lived in Alberta for five years, where in the winter time it gets cold—I mean cold. The worst I experienced was a snow storm with heavy winds, where the temperature dropped to -60°C, or -76°F. When going outside, it was necessary to ensure no skin was exposed at all. We put on many layers of clothing, gloves, goggles, a face cover, hats, and many layers of socks with heavy duty boots. It was crazy, but kind of fun for a minute.

Unfortunately, some people suffered tremendously, many froze to death, and many others ended up with serious frostbite where they lost fingers, toes, noses, or entire limbs. Some spent the entire winter complaining about how cold it was, content to be totally miserable for months on end. But, many Alberta residents have a very different way of looking at their winters. I knew a lot of people who look forward to the winter coming all year. The minute the snow finally hits, they layer up, organize themselves, grab their ski and snowboard gear, jump on a snowmobile, attach chains to their truck tires, or partake in some sort of crazy experience. They get out to have as much excitement and fun as possible in the snow.

What was the difference between these two groups of people? Perception. If you sit around looking at what bugs you, what you don't like, and have a bad mental state about anything, that's the experience you will have—bad! This will be true for as long as you hold those thoughts and feelings. But the reality is, your thoughts and feelings, your perception, can change as fast as turning on a light switch. How you choose to perceive anything is how you experience life. With using this example, I am in no way discounting or belittling countless ailments and issues that many suffer with, or saying ailment and illness is all in the mind. But, the mind and the beliefs an individual lives by, beliefs that are often very strongly held onto, do play a very important role. Change your perception and you will change your experiences, which will change your thoughts and feelings, which will change your choices, which will change your life.

The Power of the Mind

What I've learned through my studies and over 32 years of working with chronically ill people with cancer (and numerous other problems), is that the ones who want to get to the core of their own life issues and become true to themselves are generally better equipped to beat the failures, disappointments, ailments, and disease. Tragically, people who don't want to think about why they've got to a place in life that feels miserable and overwhelming tend to put their health wholly and blindly in the hands of doctors or specialists. People who believe that they are sick because of someone or something else—"it's in the genes," "it runs in the family," "there is no cure," "I was told that this was going to kill me," and so on—often remain stuck or get worse. These beliefs and this mental state are exactly what creates the perfect mental and physical environment to end up dealing with ailments for the rest of their lives, or even dying from them.

I'll rephrase that. People don't generally die from cancer; they just die. Very rarely do people die from actual cancer. They usually die from the toxicity of "treatments" and drug therapy given to them. Most conventional treatments impair a person's immune system and create inflammation. Inflammation is a leading cause to many ailments, illnesses, and diseases.[6] What's supposed to make them better actually makes them sicker.

Most times during the excessive drug "therapy" overload, the patient is instructed to stay in a dark room with no natural sunlight (because the sun is bad for you) and told not to exercise. They are left focusing on how sick they are and how crappy their life is. They're fed high-sugar foods like ice cream and jelly, which have ingredients commonly known to cause cancer in the first place. The air in the room is generally stuffy, recycled air, and the windows are kept closed to keep all that fresh air out. There is no room for laughter and joy, and eventually the body just gives up. Their attitude and mental state negatively affect their physical health, and vice versa.

Drug overdoses are also common among cancer patients, as are pneumonia and heart failure. Often people are dying because they just don't want to continue living this way any longer; giving up is just easier and less painful. They lose the ability to take responsibility for their reality, their willingness and desire to keep trying, and the energy to make a change. It becomes easier to give up than to face the hard truth that they're ultimately responsible for where they're at. (Children born with cancer and other ailments are obviously suffering for different reasons, but that's another book.)

I strongly believe illness, disease, pain, and suffering are the direct result of what we have internally created. Your beliefs about yourself and your life, your attitude, and the choices you make based on our upbringing and conditioning create what you experience. If you are

---

[6] Hunter, P. (2012). The inflammation theory of disease. *EMBO reports*, 13(11), 968-970.

suffering—emotionally, physically, or mentally, then I invite you to look at how you are its source.

It's a hard pill to swallow when we realize we no longer have anyone or anything to lay our blame upon. Often times, we are the creators of our own despair.

The good news is, we are also the healers of our own despair.

Why We Get Sick

So why do we get sick?

Besides whatever we were born with due to the environment and lifestyle choices of our parents and the environment we grew up in, the very route to our wellness lies in our emotional and mental beliefs, and in the choices we make every day. Thinking really can kill you. No thought is free of emotional implications. How we perceive what happens to us will determine whether these emotions will be stored and registered in the physical body and the reality of our personal world. "What you can see and believe, you can achieve." The truth is, both positive and negative actions and reactions can affect every aspect of your life and health.

Dr. Larry Dossey, a former internist and renowned speaker on health, believed in the power of the mind and emotions to affect health. He looked at so-called "Black Monday Syndrome," which refers to the high rate of illness and heart attacks that tend to cluster on Monday mornings at the beginning of the workweek. Dr. Dossey knew that these deaths were being caused by more than just simple stress. His work pointed out that most people with stressful jobs don't have heart attacks and many of them never even get sick. Instead, he found that Black Monday Syndrome was caused by people's attitudes they bring to work with them.

There are numbers of cases where patients have cured themselves or made impressive improvements on belief and faith alone after being given a placebo drug (a neutral substance, often a sugar pill given to someone under the pretense of it being a drug to help with a real condition). Likewise, similar patients died once that belief was taken away. The placebo effect shows the true power of the mind. If you believe you can get better, you can. If an individual believes they must live with an ailment or die from it . . . sadly, they are also often right.

I am not saying that you can wish upon a star and heal yourself, but I am also not saying that it isn't possible, either. The "amazing" and "miraculously healed" clients I have seen around the world and have been blessed to work with all changed their destiny by choice. They become very aware of how their beliefs, choices, environment, people they shared their time with, and their lifestyle was killing them. The first step was awareness. The next step for them was choosing to take the actions needed in order to change it all, and then to keep doing it.

> No matter what the "specialists" or anyone else says, you only fail when you stop and accept what they tell you at face value as a fact.

Remember, sometimes it's okay to ask for help. Asking for help means you are being courageous and strong, not weak. You are much stronger then you think you are. You are strong enough and open enough to understand that if you are feeling or living in a way that makes you feel bad or weak, it's time for a change. When you become aware of the importance of choice and change, you become strong enough to take the tiny steps towards what you know you deserve. Allow yourself time to repair, recharge, and reflect. Sometimes the most incredible things come from what seems to be an impossible challenge.

The wise Nelson Mandela stated, "It seems impossible until it is done." I bet you personally have proven this countless times, so don't stop now. Live life to the fullest. Don't limit yourself or what you are able to achieve. Stop listening to and surrounding yourself with negative people. Be true to you and the world will be yours.

Next, we'll look in greater depth at how our thinking affects the rest of our life and health.

The Importance of Mindset and Belief

There seems to be a bridge missing for people to help them make the leap to understanding how their own choices, thoughts and emotions can be at the core of their physical condition. No one said it is an easy thing to look in the mirror, especially when we have created a reality that may not reflect who we really are or what we really want.

Words and beliefs are very powerful. What are we taking away from ourselves, our children, and our friends and family if we don't open our minds? We need to look beyond the "norm" and allow new perceptions, new beliefs, and new understandings. We must allow ourselves to be guided and supported to be the best we can be and encourage others to be the best they can be to eliminate what is at the core of all the ailments and illnesses.

The job of healers, specialists and doctors is to empower, uplift, support, encourage and sometimes upset their clients to create the awareness that anything is possible and that *they* are in control. Pushing the lines of beliefs and your comfort zone is where the magic happens. We all have amazing abilities; *so many people around the world have proven this with endless success stories and "miracles."* All you need to do is allow the endless positive opportunities to come into your mind, body, and life. I'm not saying believe everything. I am saying to believe in the opportunity that anything could be possible.

No matter what the "specialists" or anyone else says, you only fail when you stop and accept what they tell you at face value as a fact. My clients and millions of others around the world have continually proven this through their own achievements that anything is possible, and the human body and mind are amazing. Believe in yourself, and keep proving them all wrong. Stay focused and stay positive. Ignore the negativity and fear from others and your own mind. Continually work towards regaining your power and achieving your goals, whatever they may be.

It isn't a stretch for most people to believe that choices, emotions, and thoughts are key players in a person's health and the creation of or recovery from an illness. Even so, when the same people are faced with issues in their own lives, they seem to throw all this wisdom out the window. Instead, they spend their time thinking about the hard blow that life has dealt them. They go off looking for external answers, embarking upon a confusing journey through the merry-go-round of pills, potions, counseling, self-help gurus, guides, group therapies, fad diets, and endless medical treatments and amazing trips, along with listening to everyone with an opinion.

You know how important it is to have the right mindset and the right attitude. You know that if you can keep your positive attitude, anything is possible. Now it comes down to training yourself to stay positive in the face of setbacks. Remind yourself that you are in control of your destiny, and stay focused on getting better. You can overcome the ailments in your life. Practice cultivating positivity in your life, and remember that your beliefs and attitude will either keep you well or make you sick. When you stay positive, you will live a naturally healthier, happier life.

The Effects of Energy

My experience with cancer patients has shown that years of not being true to yourself, bad choices, stressful lifestyles, negative energy and people, hazardous environments, and poor eating habits create energy blocks in the body. (*These blocks can even form in babies, due to the emotions and lifestyle choices of the parents.*) The blocks can disrupt the body's frequency and temperature, creating the perfect environment for cancer or other illnesses.

To understand a block in the body, imagine ice in a garden hose. (Again, coming from Canada, I have experienced this a lot.) Let's say you have a garden hose lying outside. It gets cold overnight and the water in the hose freezes. You wake up in the morning when the sun comes up and it's starting to warm up. You go outside with the sunrise and want to water your garden. You squeeze the spray nozzle and nothing comes out, or just a very small stream of water drips out.

> **Our bodies are constantly working to keep things flowing smoothly, but sometimes they need help.**

You go to check that the water main is turned on and see that it is. There is a lot of water at the main, but very little, if any, is coming out the end of the hose. Why? Because throughout the hose, the water is frozen, blocking the flow of more water through the hose. So, what do you do? Say the hose is no good anymore and throw it in the garbage? No. You move the hose around, bend it, step on it, and eventually the water starts flowing out of the hose normally.

Your body is just like that garden hose. Its energy can get blocked for many different reasons. This is often why when an individual who is chronically 'suffering from' or 'dealing with' something, even after spending a lot of time and money on products and potions, along with many tests done by countless different "specialists," is often told, "the test came back 'normal.' There's nothing wrong with you." But, you know something is wrong.

Our bodies are constantly working to keep things flowing smoothly, but sometimes they need help. When we clear the blockages, remove the negativity, and increase the energy vibration in the body, we let our immune systems send out signals to kill off invading cells. Researchers in California with cancer patients used special heating devices to raise the body temperature. The results showed success in slowing tumor growth and releasing emotional blocks from the body to restore balance and energy.

If you're going to restore balance and energy in your body, you must recognize, deal with, and release emotional blocks. Abundant scientific evidence shows that the immune system is directly compromised by emotions and thoughts, and vice versa.[7] Stress and other negative emotions suppress the immune system, making us get sick more often, and putting us at greater risk of coming down with chronic diseases and ailments. When you let go of all of that emotional baggage, you're also directly improving your health.

In a 1997 article called *Why We Get Sick*, immunologist Candace Pert identified a group of molecules called neuropeptides.[8] She believes these are the biochemicals of negative emotions. Change your beliefs, change your perception, change your environment, change your thoughts, and you will change your body and how you experience life. What is interesting about Pert's research is that every peptide she uncovered is produced both in the brain and the body. What this means, according to her, is that the emotions that we have traditionally associated with our heads live in our bodies too.

Your emotions can have a huge effect on your risk of developing life-threatening diseases, too. Alastair Cunningham, a senior scientist at the Ontario Cancer Institute in Toronto, Canada, has treated cancer by teaching people how to get in touch with their feelings. He believes emotions play a crucial role in the spread of cancer. Through his

---

[7] Dantzer, R., O'Connor, J. C., Freund, G. G., Johnson, R. W., & Kelley, K. W. (2008). From inflammation to sickness and depression: when the immune system subjugates the brain. *Nature reviews neuroscience*, 9(1), 46-56.

[8] Pert, C. (2017). *Articles*. Retrieved from http://candacepert.com/articles/.

research, he has concluded that it seems clear that repressed emotions are one of the things that make cancer more likely.

There is now a large body of evidence that clearly shows that our mentality, feelings, and beliefs play vital roles in our health. Sadly, our society largely ignores the effects of mindset on physical health. Most doctors simply ignore this evidence, since it's easier to write a prescription than it is to dig into the emotional roots, the why's and how's of an illness. We still peg all this self-responsibility talk as "a bunch of New-Age mumbo-jumbo" or, as my Grandmother called it, "hokey pokey witchcraft stuff."

There is more to healing and understanding why we get sick than meets the eye. Perhaps we need to look a little deeper. In the following chapters, that's exactly what we will do.

Key Takeaways:

Your body needs a natural and integrated approach to living. **You are in control** and have the power to create ailment and illness or great health and happiness. The choice is yours.

Your environment, mindset, words, and beliefs have a powerful physical impact on your health and the life you live. Both positive and negative impacts on your health lay in your emotional and mental beliefs, your perceptions, and the choices you make every minute of every day.

A holistic approach is necessary if you're going to find a path toward true health, happiness, and success. You are a holistic individual— your approach to your health must be as well.

Beliefs and choices are key players in a person's health and recovery from an illness. If you want to heal quickly, you must understand and acknowledge the role of your mindset and your emotions.

"

Mind-body medicine should not be an 'alternative,' nor should complementary and integrative medicine be something doctors are not exposed to during their training.

—BERNIE SIEGEL

Alternative Medicine vs. Conventional Medicine

I've mentioned conventional medicine several times already throughout the book and you know how I feel about it. So, what are your other efficient, practical, and empowering choices to incorporate with it? Besides being very aware and incorporating all of my "10 Vital Keys" into your daily life, two primary options are "alternative medicine" and "energy medicine," which is a little more advanced. Alternative medicine uses natural methods to help treat ailments, with the intent to keep you healthy. Energy medicine combines physical and non-physical elements, explores the body's energy fields, and shows you how to shift energy to create change at a cellular level. My approach is holistic and integrates all three of the approaches you will learn in this chapter, plus a few more I have discovered along the way.

Let's begin with a look at the main differences between the first two major medical systems in widespread use in the world today, conventional and alternative medicine. Then, we'll discuss how energy medicine fits in to create the holistic-style medicine I use to help my clients become the best versions of themselves.

Conventional Medicine

Conventional medicine is based on the anatomy and physiology of the physical body. It identifies the body as heart, lungs, liver, spleen, intestines, muscle tissues, connective tissues, lymphatic channels, etc. These organs link to each other in a distinct way to form different functional systems such as the circulatory system, respiratory system, digestive system, immune system, and so on.

The difference between these organs and systems is based in the cells that they're made of. Each organ has its own unique subset of specialized cells that help it perform its function within the body. The diagnosis of a disease depends on the tissues or organs in which a problem is detected. If the disease occurs in the heart, it will be named heart disease. If found in the intestine, it's an intestinal disease. Organs are seen as distinct parts of the body, and conventional medicine rarely focuses on how they are interconnected.

This limited view prevents those in the conventional medical profession from truly understanding how heart disease could cause a pain in the front chest, or how it could affect the ear or foot. Conventional doctors don't understand how heart disease could be healed by some manipulation of the ear or the arm, or on some meridian (a term used in traditional Chinese medicine). By treating systems individually, most doctors completely miss how an imbalance in one system can affect the entire body.

> Conventional medicine has many benefits, however, it is only a small part in your big puzzle, and it certainly is not a long-term strategy.

In short, conventional medical professionals are skeptical of any other medical system that is based on different principles than their own. They powerfully state that these alternative approaches are "unscientific." So, if any disease cannot be healed by conventional doctors or delayed by an early diagnosis, patients are discouraged from seeking out other types of medicine for answers, not only by the doctors and "specialists," but often and even more powerfully, by the friends and family, due to their beliefs and understanding as taught by the mainstream media and similar outlets.

I'm not at all against conventional medicine. Conventional medicine has many benefits, which is why I team up with so many doctors and "specialists" around the world. However, it is only a small part in your big puzzle, and it certainly is not a long-term strategy. When patients feel uncomfortable and no diagnosis can be made, doctors sometimes do not know what medicine to prescribe. So, they run through a list of prescription medications, prescribing one after the other until they find one that seems to help alleviate some of the symptoms the patient is experiencing. It's like throwing a handful of darts at a dart board and hoping one or two of them stick, with no real concern or discussion about what all the "try this" treatments are actually doing to your body. (Have you ever read all the warnings on the labels for medications or treatments you've been prescribed?) What's confusing to me is that this is normal, accepted, and encouraged. But, if you tell someone to use pure, organic oil of oregano to kill infection in your body and to help eliminate inflammation, and that it has no harmful negative effects on any part of your body, and people think you're crazy.

Remedies in conventional medicine usually involve drugs, which will correspond to the symptoms of the present disease. In most cases, this approach causes endless side effects and the long-term "need to live with it" mindset. Combined with medication, often times the approach conventional doctors take is to start cutting away at the body, to remove what they can see as being the issue. Alternative medicine criticizes these kinds of remedies as invasive because there are legitimate alternative healing systems that will not damage or remove any part of the body, or let patients suffer more from the effects of the treatment or surgery.

The unfortunate thing is conventional doctors also don't have the know-how, or the freedom, to get an opinion from a doctor in alternative medicine. Apparently, conventional medicine doctors must wait until a disease presents symptoms that are strong enough that they can diagnose it. You have to wait around until you're in enough discomfort or pain for them to be able to run some tests to figure out what's going on. One downfall of conventional medicine is its apparent inability to help prevent diseases from actually occurring. (And I'm not referring to the new plans to start kids on a long-term drug therapy as soon as they are born with the hopes that they may not get something that they may possibly have the chance of getting at some point in the future.)

Now modern science is going one step further. Due to the magnificence of modern science, doctors can determine if an individual has a gene that potentially could become some sort of an ailment or disease at some point in the future. Why is this so great? According to them, once you know you have the gene, you can begin taking a lifetime supply of pharmaceuticals to avoid that disease. In some cases, you could eliminate anything that would become an issue in the future. Take Angelina Jolie as an example. Her well-publicized double mastectomy was a reaction to her discovery that she carried a gene that increased her breast cancer risk. It's a good thing my father wasn't diagnosed by one of these "specialists," since he had brain cancer.

Alternative Medicine

Alternative medicine is different from conventional medicine in several ways. The most important distinction between conventional and alternative medicine is that alternative medicine makes its diagnosis on a functional basis. That diagnosis is grounded on functionally-linked organs and tissues. These organs or tissues may or may not be linked with each other anatomically, but they absolutely affect one another.

For example, a heart is functionally linked with the small intestine and the front part of the tongue. These links are used by alternative medicine practitioners to help combat heart ailments and keep them from appearing in the first place. Compared to conventional medicine, alternative medicine's approach is like looking at the physical body from far away to see the whole picture. They can understand and apply long-distance healing techniques to heal a disease. For example, a heart problem can be remedied with a needle in the ear or arms by an experienced acupuncturist.

Energy Medicine

Energy medicine, a subset of alternative medicine, takes the functional approach a step further; it's a more advanced concept. In her 1998 book, *Energy Medicine: Balancing Your Body's Energies for Optimal Health, Joy, and Vitality,* Professor Donna Eden describes energy medicine as the thread that ties science and spirituality together. It integrates the tangible and intangible, and is a way to explain the power behind being naturally you. When your energy systems are aligned, you experience health, happiness, and success. In energy medicine, doctors do not identify where the disease is within the body. To use a spatial metaphor again, they look at our physical body from even further away than even most alternative medicine modalities.

Energy medicine is established on a very solid theoretical base stating all materials in the universe are the manifestation of energy.

This is now common knowledge. Any phenomenon in the physical world is also a reflection of energy exchange. Our feelings, our thoughts, our experience of love, hate, envy, desire and so on are now well-documented to influence the aura around our body, and around others. In some cases, I believe the energy around us contributes to the physical, mental, and emotional ailments that most people experience.

The energy related to our health can have two different properties. It can be "a good" or "a bad" energy, "high vibrational" or "low vibrational," and "positive" or "negative." The dualistic nature of our natural world is helpful for looking at health issues. As you can imagine, "bad," "low vibrational," and "negative" energy lead people to have ailments and chronic illnesses, as well as encouraging or creating many addictions and bad life choices. The goal in Energy Medicine is to raise an individual's vibration. Your energy fields can accumulate energy from the environments you spend the most time in. Have you ever spent time around someone who was complaining all the time (someone with low vibrational energy)? Ever notice how you feel after you have spent time with that person? I usually feel depleted. This is how energy works. Luckily, you have control of your vibration, and you choose who you share your time and energy with.

Energy medicine can be as simple as taking a walk-in nature when you are stressed. The good "natural" energy of the forest will raise your vibrational frequency. Choosing to eat more whole and natural foods that are filled with vitality "good" energy, and fewer processed, "bad" energy foods will contribute to good health. However, conventional doctors do not pay attention to your energy system and they don't understand its integral role it can play in a person's healing process.

With the development of energy medicine, it has become easier and more intuitive to understand the many different forms of energy healing. They are:

• Chinese acupuncture—Qigong
• Reiki—therapeutic touch
• Shamanism healing—long-distance healing
• Mind-healing—religion healing
• Light and sound therapy

Any foods, herbs, supplements, chemicals, or drugs can all be regarded as energy entities and therefore have an effect on your health. I have talked about choices. What we choose to eat and put on our bodies, who we choose to spend most of our time with, what we choose to think about and where we choose to spend our time all have an impact on our energy systems.

My approach to health offers you another level of awareness—to discover who you want to be in this lifetime and what kind of life you want to live. Is it one with pain and suffering? Boring. Or is it an extraordinary life that empowers you to be naturally you, free to love, free to be healthy and free to be and maintain the success you have always dreamed of?

Chinese and Ayurvedic Medicine

The greatest achievement in traditional Chinese medicine is its recognition of the meridian system. The Chinese found that there was life energy (*qi*) flowing through the meridians, and that *qi* is essential to our body's function. The existence of meridians was originally denied by the Western medicine system because it could not be seen or detected at that time. However, more doctors are now admitting that the meridian system can be "felt," and scientists have even illustrated these meridians with the use of radiolabeled infusions.

However, traditional Chinese medicine is not perfect either. First, there are many diseases that cannot be healed by it. Second, it does not recognize the importance of the chakra system in our body. The chakras are seven energy centers found throughout the body that were re-discovered by practitioners of Ayurvedic medicine (Indian medicine) between 1500 and 500 BC. The chakra system has been worked with and written about by the Sumerians thousands of years before, long before traditional Chinese or Ayurvedic medicine.

Modern scholars and philosophers have noted symbolic parallels to the Indian "Kundalini," a spiritual energy in the body depicted as a coiled serpent rising up from the base of the spine to the Third Eye (Pineal Gland) in the moment of enlightenment. Awakened Kundalini represents the merging and alignment of the Chakras, and is said to be the one and only way to attain the "Divine Wisdom," which brings pure joy, pure knowledge, and pure love.[1]

Third, Chinese traditional medicine does not emphasize the spiritual aspect of the occurrence and healing of a disease. That spiritual link is

---

[1] Whitaker, A. (2012, April). Ancient Wisdom: Sumeria. Retrieved from *http://www.ancient-wisdom.com/sumeria.htm*.

acknowledged by Buddhism, Hinduism, and many other religions. The alternative medical approach to healing and health encourages a relationship with spirituality and doesn't reject its role in the healing process.

Another gap I discovered in traditional Chinese medicine is that it overlooks life choices, lifestyle, environment, and stress. As I explained earlier, all these other factors play the initial and important role in the why's and how's of what is now happening in the body and what can happen in the future. Your mental outlook and your beliefs have a huge effect on your overall health, including whether or not you get sick or develop a disease.

Despite their limitations, we have much to learn from these traditional alternative medical systems. Ayurvedic medicine integrates spirituality, which has a huge effect on a patient's ability to stay healthy, or to recover from a disease or illness. The energy medicine found in a prescribed herb mixture, the most-used remedy in Chinese medicine, could positively affect a patient's recovery. Patients see results when the herbs are extracted from their active components and applied to support those patients' ailments. These alternative health systems work because they are based on ancient knowledge of our body's underlying energy pathways, pathways that connect organs and bodily systems to each other.

I believe using a combination of alternative and conventional medicine is the best approach to ultimate health, happiness, and success in treating dis-ease, pain, and chronic illness. It's the only way to see the whole picture of what's causing a patient to experience symptoms. And, it's the only way to take actions that will support the whole person and body, not just one part, or one part of the part. The body as a whole functions as the sum of its interconnected systems. Focusing on one system at a time is not an effective way to treat a patient.

In the next few sections, we'll look at a few life-changing therapies and techniques that the conventional medicine system neglects.

Migraine Therapy

Wouldn't it be great to be free of a migraine—completely—with little to no side effects?

What causes a migraine exactly is still debated by scientific researchers. The pain itself is caused by swollen blood vessels in the head, which are affected by chemical changes in the body. But what causes those chemical changes that cause the blood vessels to swell in the first place? And how can that root cause be addressed to eliminate migraine pain?

As a migraine sufferer, your priority is to learn what creates your pain, rather than masking it. Most patients who have more than two headache episodes per month, or those very much disabled by headaches, must begin a preventative therapy. Beta blockers are typically the first choice in these cases, but that's not what I recommend. Amitriptyline is also commonly used, and there seems to be a widespread use of calcium-channel blockers for "conventional" prevention of a migraine, although the benefits are controversial. Unfortunately, two of the most effective conventional medications for prevention of a migraine, methysergide and phenelzine, are usually relegated to last-resort use because of potentially serious side effects.

I work with migraine sufferers to help them naturally eliminate their symptoms. I help give control back to the sufferer. My approach eliminates the pill popping, and the side effects of taking so many medications. Many doctors would agree that many of these prescribed medications are ineffective, and when used over long periods, and when combined with other pharmaceuticals and heavily-processed foods and sugars, result in long lists of ailments and symptoms. My clients learn to live normally by making choices that enhance the best version of themselves, helping them eliminate any need to use these drugs. The treatments I support are an entirely logical approach. They are non-invasive, pain-free, and do not use any form of tablet, pill, or potion.

The method I recommend relieves the migraine by helping to restore alignment in the neck and head, along with imbalances in the organs and other areas of the body that may be causing or contributing to the migraine problem. It's important to examine your structure, work on the bones of the head, and reinvigorate the energy flow throughout the meridians and chakras in your body, while becoming aware of the foods and products you put in and on your body. In addition, your environment and the people you share your time and energy with all play a very powerful role. This usually means that my clients see an almost immediate drop in the frequency of migraine attacks after a very short period of time, in many cases, immediately.

The key to my hands-on approach is reading and feeling the body, while using various styles and techniques of massage around the skull, spine, and core, including the organs. This touching is essential and it allows me to be able to "listen" with my hands to what is called the cranial rhythmic impulse. This pulsation is distinct from both the familiar cardiovascular pulse and the normal breathing rhythm. To the experienced practitioner, this pulse has a cycle of three seconds of inflow and three seconds of rest, averaging 10 cycles per minute. When there is interruption of the inflow by abnormal restrictions, such as from an injury or by abnormal tension, the disrupted patterns may result in problems such as dizziness, migraine headaches, blurred vision, concentration problems, mood swings, and sinus problems.

Once I have identified these patterns of congestion or resistance, I then locate their cause, and I gently perform the manipulations needed. I free up the resistance and restore natural balance to the pulse. My clients experience fewer migraines because they have a more balanced structure throughout their head and neck, and the likelihood of the vasoconstriction or vasodilatation that occurs in migraines decreases. Combine the hands-on work with awareness of the environment and daily choices, and the migraines will be long forgotten.

> The key to my hands-on approach is reading and feeling the body, while using various styles and techniques of massage around the skull, spine, and core, including the organs.

This alternative treatment is safe and gentle and can be used with babies, young children, the elderly, and anyone in between. The boost in circulation means that the healing agents of the body itself are triggered into action. Fresh oxygen and nutrients are brought to your body's tissues. The natural side effects of this treatment are freedom from pain, a better attitude toward life, and the awareness that anything is possible. The body's own painkillers are being naturally released. These feel-good chemicals help to restore your health and vitality without the negative side effects of conventional medicine treatments.

Detoxification Cleansing Therapy

Another alternative treatment I believe in, and consider to be one of the keys to ultimate health, happiness, and success, is detoxing your body. Detox is a practice to support you in achieving the best version of you. But, it's important to make sure you are following the right type of detox. Being naturally you means making educated choices that serve your highest self, so choosing the latest fad may not be in your best interest.

Think of your body as being like your car, or your bike. You ensure it is regularly serviced and cared for. You probably wash it regularly, inside and out. You keep an eye on the tire, water, and oil pressure. At scheduled intervals, you get the oil changed, ensure all the liquids are clean, filled, and maintained. All the moving parts are regularly lubed, tightened, adjusted, and/or replaced when needed. Do you maintain your body with the same care and attention?

If your car were in need of an oil change, would you think it would save you time and money if instead of replacing the oil, you just put in a new oil filter, without changing the old dirty oil at the same time? What would happen to the brand-new oil filter if you did that? How long would the new oil filter last?

What would happen if you just ignored the oil altogether and just drove as far as you could, for as long as you could? How long would that engine last?

If you can imagine this, or you would never do this, why then would you do the latest "celebrity" or "fad" detox of your body, without ensuring the right system is being cleansed in the right order? If you have ever heard that a detox can be dangerous, or you have heard of someone getting sick during or after a detox, this is a sure sign that they did the wrong detox at the wrong time, and probably the wrong way.

There are many different systematic body cleansing and detoxifying programs, and I highly recommend that you work with an expert to guide you while trying out any new detox program. When you follow the right detox programs at the right time, in the right way for you and your body, the interconnected systems in your body will all come into alignment, and the results can literally be magical. Detoxifying can open the door to endless benefits, such as mental clarity, increased immunity, increased energy, healthier looking skin and hair, stronger memory, better eyesight and concentration, and oftentimes permanent weight loss because the toxic fat has been released from the body.

How do you know when to detox or cleanse? I always recommend that people consider detoxing their body and lives consistently. We live in a world where toxins are found everywhere and in everything, including the creams, lotions, perfumes, deodorants, soaps, and shampoos we slather on our skin every single day. We're exposed to toxins from the water we drink, the bed and sheets we sleep on, the air we breathe, and the foods we eat. We are literally surrounded and inundated by chemical toxins. So, it makes sense that you should be detoxing on a regular basis.

Again, think of your car, or your clothes. You don't just wash them once, then forget about it and never do it again. Depending on where you live or spend your time, you realize this is a never-ending process. I lived in London, UK for a few years, and it shocked me when I came home at night after a day in the city. I literally had dirt lines where my skin was exposed. My shirts were almost black, a very noticeable color change, especially when wearing white. When I got in the shower, the water running off me looked as though I was working in the farm yard all day. If your clothes and skin get that dirty from just a few hours out in the city, imagine what's going on inside your body day after day, month after month, year after year . . .

Another way to know when to cleanse is to look and listen to your body and the signals it's sending to you. If you notice that you:

- have low energy, you keep getting sick,
- find your focus and mental clarity become foggy,
- are experiencing mood swings,
- experience spots in your eyes, buzzing in your ears, or headaches,
- find spots or blotches on your skin or your skin is itchy,
- wake up during the night, or you sleep all night but wake up tired,
- experience indigestion and heartburn,
- have smelly breath, farts and urine, or
- crave certain types of foods and sugary treats,

. . . then it's time for a detox. Symptoms that don't feel normal to you and your life are a big indicator that it may be necessary to detox.

One of the biggest reasons I believe in cleansing is that it contributes to the optimization of your immune system. One cleanse I recommend is colon cleansing because it benefits the liver and ultimately your immune system. The immune system is your key to combating invasions of your body. Our immune system battles microorganisms that pollute our bodies, resulting in ailments. When our immune systems have been weakened, we jeopardize our health, happiness, and success. Detoxifying protects and promotes the healing process.

If our body cannot detoxify properly, the consequence is a disease. If your body isn't cleansing and detoxing itself properly, you'll start to experience all sorts of health problems. We can't heal ourselves without cleansing the intestines because intestinal function is strongly tied to immune function. That's why eliminating toxins from our systems using a detox therapy is a major key to healing from the inside out.

A proper colon detox will also help to maintain a healthy digestive system, which has a huge impact on how you feel overall. Studies have proven that if you seem deficient in the proper nutrients that your body needs, it may be because your intestines are not absorbing them properly.[234] Detoxing will help clean your intestines so they can absorb nutrients from the food you eat more efficiently. (Think of a dirty sponge or a clogged drain. If the stuff can't get through, your body can't use it, no matter how great your nutritional intake is.) When your body gets the nutrients it needs, your immune system will function as it was meant to, and you will become and stay healthy.

Symptoms of Colon Dysfunction

Many of the symptoms patients commonly complain about are actually due to the colon not working like it's supposed to. This partial list of symptoms connected with colon dysfunction is freely available on the Internet. However, it is how you *use* this information and our programs to eradicate them that makes the difference.

appetite loss	gastritis	inflammation
asthma	hemorrhoids	parasite infections
backaches	hypoglycemia	prostate problems
bad breath	hyperactive activity	respiratory ailments
cancer	immune dysfunction	short attention span
cirrhosis of the liver	impotence	skin problems
colitis	indigestion	swollen stomach
concentration loss	insomnia	tension
congestion	irritability	toxic feeling
digestive disorders	learning difficulties	urinary disorders
distended abdomen	nail fungus	vaginitis
food craving	nervousness	weight problems
foul gas	pancreatitis	yeast infection

[2] James, W. P. T. (1968). Intestinal absorption in protein-calorie malnutrition. *The Lancet*, 291(7538), 333-335.

[3] Arroyave, G., Viteri, F., Béhar, M., & Scrimshaw, N. S. (1959). Impairment of intestinal absorption of vitamin A palmitate in severe protein malnutrition (kwashiorkor). *The American journal of clinical nutrition*, 7(2), 185-190.

[4] Wapnir, R. A. (2000). Zinc deficiency, malnutrition and the gastrointestinal tract. *The Journal of nutrition*, 130(5), 1388S-1392S.

That's a huge list of symptoms, but it doesn't even come close to the full list! I'm sure you're beginning to understand the importance of colon health, and how taking care of your colon can help you feel better in your body. One of the ways to support colon health is with a colon cleanse. Benefits of colon cleansing and detoxification therapy are:

- Clearing blockages
- Cleaning the blood
- Preventing the production of gallstones
- Breaking down cholesterol
- Clearing up yeast and parasite infections
- Stopping inflammation
- Controlling blood pressure
- Restoring pH balance
- Improving digestion and all the other symptoms previously mentioned.

So how does a colon cleanse and detox work? To learn how this specialized detoxification process helps your colon, it's important to remember that all of your body's organs and systems are interconnected. By supporting the health of organs like your liver and pancreas, you're actually supporting your colon health, too.

The liver is one of the most important organs in the body. The liver performs over 500 functions. Along with filtering out toxins and producing bile for digestion, it is the filter that regulates the levels of good and bad chemicals. The liver is a part of the biliary system, which consists of the liver, gallbladder, pancreas, and duodenum.

One of the important functions of your liver is to produce bile, which then is used in digestion and other essential processes in your body. The liver produces bile in its polygonal cells from cholesterol (bilirubin and biliverdin) and bile salts (acids), which are linked from the amino acids' glycine, glycolic, taurine, and taurocholic acid. From the liver, bile travels through the hepatic duct, where it connects to the common bile duct and the cystic duct. The bile travels up the bile duct to be stored in the gallbladder. When bile is needed during digestion, it travels into the common bile duct through the ampulla and enters the duodenum, a section of the small intestine.

The pancreas is another important part of the biliary system. Among other things like insulin, the pancreas also produces lipase. Lipase is an enzyme which increases the production of the hormones that stimulate contractions of the gall bladder while fats are being digested. This causes the opening of the ampulla so bile can flow into the duodenum. So, the pancreas, liver, and gall bladder all work in tandem to help your body digest food efficiently.

When the biliary system is functioning properly, all the other organs can perform their job more efficiently. When it self-cleans, the waste and poisons that have been absorbed from the blood are rendered as harmless compounds ready for elimination. If the passage has not been cleared, waste and poisons accumulate and sit around in your body, affecting all the other organs and systems.

Cleansing stimulates the release of bile. Detox therapies stimulate the release of hepatic bile and promote healing. When more bile is released, more toxins can be broken down in the small intestine. And, the increased bile production also helps clear out the liver as well. Flushing out accumulated toxins and debris in the liver allows the biliary system to absorb better and do its job.

If you're experiencing symptoms of colon dysfunction, don't wait to fix the problem. The longer you wait, the more your condition deteriorates. Degeneration and deterioration come about slowly. Life goes on without our noticing that we have a serious problem until it happens. We often hear how, "Everything was great and then just suddenly something happened." Well, it almost never actually happens suddenly. Most of the times the small signs were ignored; even many of the bigger signs are often ignored, or masked by popping some sort of pill or potion. So, the body decided to send a more extreme signal that it's time to do some maintenance. Something alarming or a serious health problem occurs because we didn't pay attention to the smaller alarms. Intestinal dysfunction is one of those small alarms. If ignored, it will be followed by bigger ones, which are far more serious and will take longer to reverse.

If your large intestine is at least partially clear, you can concentrate on cleansing your small intestine. It is just as important, as it helps the self-detox to function. Self-irrigation will help regulate your bowel movements and restore your intestinal muscle tone, which normalizes muscular contractions (peristalsis). Peristalsis stimulates your liver, helping it to produce bile. These muscle contractions also help in absorbing lipids and fat-soluble vitamins into the body. The absorption of nutrients is also higher if the large intestine is clean. All the above strategies help your body heal faster and rejuvenate more quickly.

WARNING: As everyone is unique and each situation is different, I design each program specifically for the client and his or her individual needs. Be very careful when considering any detoxification therapy, as there are many websites and products available to do it yourself. There are no shortcuts to health and there is no such thing as a cookie-cutter program that works for everyone. You are an individual and everything about you, your body, and your lifestyle needs to be taken into consideration *before* embarking on any sort of detoxification or cleansing program.

Later in the book you will find more about detoxifying your life. I will talk about how detoxifying your home and work environments dramatically affect the life you are creating for yourself. When you follow the suggestions in this book, you will experience the control and power you have over your health, and you'll see the powerful effects that tiny steps and different choices make in all aspects of your life. The key, and fun part of this journey, will be to explore and create a program that is best for you, so as to achieve and maintain the lifestyle you are designing for yourself. Find what works for you through creating your own individualized program that brings you the results you have always wanted. But don't worry; I'll be here to guide you through the process as much as I can in the book, and if you wish, my team or I can support you personally.

My Beliefs on It All

Through my decades of experience and training I have come to understand none of the different types of "medicine" or "healing techniques" on their own will work effectively or completely in the long term. It's important to know that focusing on only one or a couple different aspects of the individual is not supportive to a person's overall health, happiness, and success. All the interconnectedness of our systems needs to be managed and supported together and at the same time, or at least you need to be aware of how all is connected. As I always say, "it's never just one thing" and "everything affects and effects everything."

I offer you a different approach from a different viewpoint. My approach is different from the 'normal' systems that are generally used throughout the world today. Although my approach can and should be used in conjunction

ALTERNATIVE MEDICINE VS CONVENTIONAL MEDICINE
I believe using a combination of alternative and conventional
medicine is the best approach to ultimate health, happiness,
and success in treating dis-ease, pain, and chronic illness.

CONVENTIONAL BASED MEDICINE
Disease Oriented, Doctor Centered

CHINESE & AYURVEDIC MEDICINES
Based on Ancient Knowledge of Underlying Energy Pathways

REG'S 10 VITAL KEYS

ALTERNATIVE MEDICINE
Health Oriented, Patient Centered

ENERGY MEDICINE
Based on Energy and Vibrational Frequency,

with modern medicine, awareness, and common sense, the 'magic' and
extraordinary living that results from my approach comes from the ten keys
that provide real life strategies to greater amounts of passion, prosperity,
health, wealth, happiness, and success in *all* areas of your life. Grasp the ten
keys to clearly understand this message. It's all about the choices you will
make once you have a new awareness, and the steps you will take to achieve
and maintain the powerful and extraordinary life you love.

Key Takeaways:

Achieving your "Ultimate Life," truly living the life where you can naturally "BE YOU," needs to occur through a combination of approaches, i.e., the holistic approach. There are three main approaches to healing illness and disease: conventional, alternative, and energy medicine.

Conventional medicine is based on the anatomy of the physical body and relies largely on reactive medicine, treatment, and pharmaceuticals. Doctors trained in traditional medicine generally focus on treating symptoms the patient is experiencing.

Alternative medicine focuses on the functionality of the "whole" body including organs and tissues. Traditional Chinese medicine and Ayurvedic (Indian) medicine are two of the ancient medical systems that serve to support a natural healing approach to the physical body and its health and happiness.

Energy medicine shows us that to heal your body, bad energy must be replaced with good energy. Replacing low vibrational energy with high vibrational energy can help you feel better, both physically and mentally, as well as support you in making the right choices. Look for an acupuncturist, Reiki master, and sound healer to incorporate energy healing in your everyday life, while being very aware of how you feel when you are around different people, and are in different environments.

The "10 Vital Keys" bring everything together! My intention is to create awareness of HOW the lifestyle, people, environments, products, foods, activities, and choices you make positively or negatively control and affect your health, happiness, and success, as well as your 'Brand Value.' The choices you make every minute of every day due to your beliefs ensure you are living the life you love, and loving the life you live long term, or not. It is equally as important to clearly understand WHY the body and mentality you experience everything in directly affects what you can achieve and maintain in all aspects of your life.

"

It's choice —
not chance — that
determines your
destiny.

—JEAN NIDETCH

Your Body, Your Choice!

O ne of the most powerful—and one of the scariest—things to learn is that you are in total control of your life. The fact is, you don't *have* to live with negativity, ailments and pain. Each day, you make choices that will either positively or negatively impact your health and your life. You are in total control of your health and how you feel. One of the biggest choices you will make when it comes to your health is what advice you will actually integrate into your life.

Your body, mind, emotions, and attitude are all highly affected, either positively or negatively, by whatever and whomever you habitually choose to put into, onto, and around your body. The severity of the effects of what you put in and on your body absolutely varies. Someone who ingests too much arsenic dies within minutes, yet believe it or not, arsenic is allowed and intentionally put into products that are legally sold and widely used these days. So, if a lot kills you, what are little bits regularly doing to you?

More commonly, children often get hyperactive soon after eating something sugary, and then they're labeled with ADD or some other diagnosis. Do you see the connection? Or, think how you feel after you have come home from a long, stressful day at work and pour yourself a good, stiff drink. What about those lonely, depressing nights filled with ice cream and chocolate? These are all examples of how the food or substances we put in our bodies can affect our thoughts, feelings, energy level, and health almost immediately, and how we feel mentally or physically after it all wears off.

None of these effects is a coincidence, and none of this should be taken lightly. There's a reason why the phrase, "You are what you eat" has been repeated over and over for centuries. If you want to feel great, both physically and mentally, you need to *choose* to put the right things in and on your body. When you are putting good, 'earthy,' nutritious foods and substances into and onto your body, you are choosing to support a healthier, happier, more naturally-energized you. So, the reality is, it's not really the 'how much' of what you're eating; it's just the 'what'. This is why fad diets and calorie counting generally doesn't work. Consuming mainly processed and genetically-modified foods full of synthetic chemicals is poisoning your body, as are many of the products you put on you and around you. But, they do it much more slowly than arsenic. And, more immediately, those processed foods and products will affect you mentally and physically, which then of course affects every other aspect of your life and performance. They may make you feel great at first, full of energy or happier, but in a period of time, those exact same foods will make you feel sluggish, tired, and even depressed.

Why is what you put in, on, and around you so important? Calories are calories, right? *Wrong!* You've probably heard people say, "Your body is a furnace. It just burns up whatever foods you put into it." Do you believe that? The idea that you can eat, drink, or use whatever you want, whenever you want, without being aware of its nutritional and energetic value, is complete nonsense. It all most definitely directly affects whether you can maintain high levels of mental and physical performance, or even achieve and maintain really good health, happiness, and success long term.

Eventually, poor choices catch up with everyone. One of my favorite people used to always say, "everyone has a different shelf life." Even those skinny kids in college who eat junk but don't put on any extra weight eventually pay the price, one way or another. As they get older, the effects of their poor choices and habits build up in their bodily systems. They eventually either get fat and sluggish or grow into "sick skinny people," who seem healthy on the surface, but who have compromised immune systems, low energy levels, and other health issues. (You know, those people who looked so healthy and 'all of a sudden' some terrible health issue arose.). And, down the road, those people who have poor lifestyle habits, who eat lots of processed foods, use low energy products, don't get the right quality of sleep, push themselves too hard, and force themselves to be in negative environments or around negative people, are at a higher risk of developing all sorts of chronic ailments, illnesses and issues, like low energy, sleep problems, weight concerns, depression, aches, pains, diabetes, heart disease, cancer, dementia, and so much more. This all affects how happy, productive and successful you will be in all aspects of your life.

Your body needs the 'earthy' stuff for its fuel It is vital! Your body needs whole, minimally-processed foods to function properly. When you eat the right food, use natural products, and share your time with the right people in the right environments, you're helping your body stay in tune naturally. It responds to energy, vibration, and rhythms—and it lives in its own rhythms due to everything in, on, and around it. The rhythms of the day-and-night cycle, the weather conditions, movement, emotions, choices, beliefs, and the electrochemical charges generated by your thoughts and perception all directly and drastically affect you. Your body responds to "energy." Your body even responds to potential threats to health with its immune system. The strength and efficiency of your immune system is directly affected by every aspect of your lifestyle choices, thoughts, beliefs, and feelings.

The Power of Choice

Still not convinced that your beliefs and choices are the most powerful tools you have to change your life? Let me give you an example of the power of choice from my own story. Rather than sticking to my initial choice of becoming a medical doctor, following along a path that just didn't feel right to me, I chose to make a change and to venture out on my own journey that brought me through a very different and difficult road of discovery. That choice ultimately empowered me with the passion I have dedicated my life to. That choice, even in the face of misunderstanding, negativity, belittlement, and sarcastic judgment, has helped me to create my own 'Ultimate Life', while I am learning to "BE ME" in the life I love.

My choice has encouraged me to support myself and others through the how's of taking responsibility, and learning to live an exceptional life. My choice has blessed me with endless positive experiences, including the very exciting and powerful experiences of being there when a client has proven all the "specialists" wrong. This choice has allowed me to help thousands of clients live better, healthier, happier, and more successful lives by finding a solution to the underlying problem that was creating the symptoms arising in the body and mind. We got to the core of the issue and eliminated it, rather than continuing to help them maintain a low level of contentment, while coping with, "managing" or dying from, that unhealthy, unhappy, and unsuccessful lifestyle.

Here's another example: Natalie is a 37-year-old stay-at-home mom. She was tired all the time, which of course affected the relationship she had with her husband and children. But, she just assumed that was 'normal' and inevitable when she spent almost all of her day chasing after her three kids and maintaining the home. She didn't realize how the choices she was making were affecting every aspect of her life and the lives of her children. Every day, she was drinking at least six cups of coffee, plus a couple energy drinks to help give her the power she needed, and she was relying on processed, sugar-laden fast and 'easy' foods to help perk her up, too. She didn't understand that the food, coffee, and sugar were only giving her mood a temporary boost, and that she'd experience an even bigger crash and more harmful effects later. She also didn't realize that eating and drinking all of that sugar and caffeine could lead to major chronic health issues down the road, even though she was at a healthy weight now.

Natalie was also very surprised when we discussed how she was feeding her children. She was brought up to believe giving her kids a "treat" regularly and feeding them three meals a day plus snacks was good for them. When we sat down and took a look at all the foods she was buying, it almost all came from the center isles in the grocery store. She believed those foods were saving her time and money and making the children happy. She also was under the belief that her children "deserved a nice or fun treat every once in a while."

The reality is quite the opposite! All these little processed and sugary treats she was giving her children to "keep them happy" were creating the wild and crazy house they were living in, which was a big part of her energy drain. And, it was also costing her a lot of time and money with doctors and "specialists" due to all health issues, labels, and symptoms the children were dealing with on a regular basis. All the sugar and processed foods, as well as the environment they were all living in, drastically affected those little bodies and minds. She was shocked when we put it all down on paper to add up the actual cost of time, money, and energy needed to maintain this lifestyle!

The two older children were also both on a variety of pharmaceuticals and 'natural health products' to help deal with their many issues. When we added up all the time, money, and energy wasted running around to "specialists" trying to figure out why the children act the way they do and why they have all the health issues they do, plus all the time and money it took to research and buy either pharmaceuticals or 'healthy' products to counteract all the issues, it became very clear. Feeding children with the 'cheap' and 'easy' processed foods and sugary 'treats' actually cost far more time, money, and energy than buying high-quality, great-tasting organic and natural foods. It also cost more than educating them about the importance of taking care of their bodies, minds, and environment ever could. And remember, the way you feed and educate your children when they are small will absolutely and dramatically impact their health, happiness, and success throughout their entire adulthood, as well as how they will guide their own children.

Another very key point was their environment. Everything affects everything. (Have I mentioned that before?) It wasn't only the processed foods and sugary treats that were creating so many disruptions in their home. How the home was organized, arranged, decorated, and displayed was creating its own set of negative issues. We also studied the air and water quality in the home, the toxic off-gassing from the new beds they bought for the children, and many of their toys, along with the 'energy affecting elements,' such as; electrical, radio and Wi-Fi, and found they were all causing physical and emotional complications. The harsh laundry detergents the family used on their towels, sheets, and clothing, along with the fun and sparkly bubble baths, toothpastes, and hair gels were all contributing to the children's problems, too. All of these things together ensured these children's bodies and minds were in full-on confusion, protection, repair, and hyperactivity mode all the time. They were full of "fight and flight" energy.

Together, Natalie and I stepped though some very easy-to-implement tweaks and adjustments in the home, which immediately changed the way the house felt and the children behaved. Switching to a nutritional intake based on eating lots of fun and great-tasting natural foods gave Natalie a massive, natural energy boost, which lasted all day. She even cut out her coffee and energy drinks all together.

The children were almost instantly calmer and happier naturally, without drugs! For free! Everyone's mood has improved and as she put it, "our home environment is a much happier place to be!" She no longer snaps at her kids like she used to when she was feeling tired and overwhelmed, and they were no longer "battling a war with each other."

Rather than spending their days running around to different "specialists" or researching and buying more products, the family was now enjoying their time together making their own household and personal products and fun foods and treats that "taste way better than the other stuff." Plus, Natalie's relationship with her husband is "so much better" because she's happier overall, and she has more energy to share with him at the end of the day after the kids go to bed. Her choice to improve the home environment, make smart family choices, and put better food and products in and on her family's bodies helped her to change all of their lives, now and in the future. Even the teachers and the doctors of the two older children "are amazed with the change!"

How many people do you know who are living a "healthy lifestyle" but are constantly tired, unhealthy or overweight? I personally know so many "professionals" in multiple fields of health and wellbeing who are always getting the latest cold going around. They spend most of their days feeling cranky, stressed out, or depressed. Many of these people have bad relationships, unbalanced health, uncontrollable mood swings, and are not able to maintain high levels of health and success long term—or once they achieve a high level of success, they quickly lose it. Most people who think they're following a healthy lifestyle really aren't when you look at it closely.

When we look around us today, we see a lot of people who are complaining about aches and pains, so many that it's almost become normalized. I meet people daily who tell me nothing is wrong and they are "fine." Then, when we start to talk more, the lists of minor ailments, issues, concerns, and problems become seemingly endless. This should not be normal, but in today's world, it is. I want to shed a bright light on the issue because I know in my core that this is not how we should live. Surviving is not living an extraordinary life. You deserve that extraordinary life.

It's so clear to me how the choices we make every day affect every aspect of our lives, including health, happiness, relationships, careers, and successes. It always surprises me when I witness an individual who has no idea that they're suffering a difficult life as a direct result of how they are choosing to live life. They know it's not the kind of life they wanted for themselves. No one wants a life where they continually suffer from ailment and illness while feeling sad, unfulfilled, and maybe a bit lost. No one wants to continually fail in their career, and end up in the wrong relationships over and over again.

So why do so many find themselves in these situations? Simply put, they are ignoring the cause of their issues while spending endless amounts of time and money to maintain their beliefs and a lifestyle that they've been told they should want, or need to learn to live with.

The reality is, sometimes it starts with a single choice. For example, I chose to get out of the dream, created by the belief that becoming a 'Doctor' was the only way to fulfill my yearning to learn and help others, and to make enough money to live the lifestyle I wanted. That choice, which only took an instant, dramatically changed my life. That very scary, confusing and controversial choice would become my life's passion. You can choose to ask the deeper questions about the sources of unhappiness and suffering in your life. But, even more importantly, you must want to hear and apply the answers. When things don't "feel" right, it's time to pay attention and make a change. You are in charge of your life. You have the power to make it better—or worse—it is your choice.

Lobsters and Salmon

While waiting in an office one day I came across an article written by Eda LeShan, "How Do Lobsters Grow?"[1] This became one of my favorite short stories, because I believe it can help you understand the importance of choice and change. The title of the story posed a great question: how do lobsters, soft animals that live inside a hard, inflexible shell, grow bigger? The short story went on to explain that the only way growth is possible "is for the lobster to shed its shell at regular intervals. When its body begins to feel cramped inside the shell, the lobster instinctively looks for a reasonably safe spot to rest while the hard shell comes off and the pink membrane just inside forms the basis of the next shell. But no matter where a lobster goes for this shedding

---

[1] LeShan, E. J. (1981). The Risk of Growing. Woman's Day Magazine.

process, it is very vulnerable. It can get tossed against a coral reef or eaten by a fish. In other words, a lobster has to risk its life to grow."

After reading Eda's article, I found myself preoccupied with the lobster story for days. This story shows that life can be overwhelming, isolating and depressing because we are feeling confined and stuck by our circumstances which we have created. In that moment, I recognized that this reflected my life and the lives of many people I know and have worked with. What does the lobster do? The lobster takes time out to make the change it must go through by hiding under a rock formation to protect it from predators. During this 'me time,' it sheds its shell. It then produces a larger, stronger, and more spacious shell that allows it to grow. However, as the lobster grows, this new shell eventually becomes too confining again, so the lobster repeats the process. Off with the restricting shell, which is harder and more difficult to remove each time, to allow for a more spacious and stronger one. This process is repeated until the lobster reaches its maximum size.

While visualizing this process, I realized that discomfort is what causes the lobster to shed the shell that it is outgrowing. I looked at how humans deal with discomfort and imagined what would happen if a lobster had access to a doctor or "specialist." I bet the lobster would complain of discomfort and get a prescription for a pill, or it would be offered some medical or magical procedure to treat its symptoms. It may even sit around for years talking about how uncomfortable its life is, and has been for a long time. With the discomfort gone, or rather 'managed,' the lobster would never grow out of its shell, keeping it confined and uncomfortable. Eventually, it would die as a tiny, unfulfilled lobster.

In our modern world of "this is normal" and "you need to take something" or the latest "quick fix solutions," we are creating bigger cultural issues by encouraging people to look outward, to try endless ways to relieve discomfort, or to continue to live in a life that just doesn't fulfill who they really are, what they want, or what they need. Do you think this approach to wellness and healing is in your best interest? Do you think taking a medication (or even having a drink, or whatever) every time something is uncomfortable or difficult will help you become a better, happier person? My big question is: should every discomfort be eliminated by a pill, medical procedure, or psychological diagnosis?

The discomfort we feel might be the mind or body's way of signaling to us that we need to look at what is going on in ourselves and our lives.

It is our guide to support us in our growth and transformation, while also guiding us to discovering our natural path to truly "Be You!" Our psychological and physical discomfort can lead us into or out of being the best natural version of ourselves possible. When we know and really believe that we can change, get unstuck, and feel good about ourselves and our lives, everything changes! We can make the choice to implement the right actions consistently, and do this repeatedly throughout our lives, just like the lobster in Eda's short story.

Yes, I am aware that there may be some physical and psychiatric conditions that do require medication, but our modern world has become accustomed to taking a pill or finding immediate relief from every pain and discomfort in the body and mind. In addition, there are hundreds of scientific studies showing the benefits of simply turning inward. For example, exercise, detoxing the body, going for a walk, taking a course to enrich the mind, meditation, doing things to help others, getting a pet, as well as all the things we have already covered, such as changing your environment and becoming aware of the foods and products you use, have all been shown to help improve mild to extreme depression, anxiety, as well as other ailments and illnesses, over and over again.[2][3][4]

Our culture has created fear around being uncomfortable or in pain, and society has become unwilling to explore discomfort as a means for growth and innovation. We actively look for ways to avoid being uncomfortable or uneasy, or we look for ways to distract ourselves from those feelings. Unfortunately, that means most people will choose to stay inside their comfort zones, staying in the relationship, keeping that J.O.B., living in that home, or in that town. They take the pills they're told to take, try all the 'options,' and have those new procedures. And, they experience all the new and thrilling opportunities so they can feel "alive" comfortably, in a managed state, safe, secure, and in

[2] Hofmann, S. G., Sawyer, A. T., Witt, A. A., & Oh, D. (2010). The effect of mindfulness-based therapy on anxiety and depression: A meta-analytic review. *Journal of consulting and clinical psychology*, 78(2), 169.

[3] Ramel, W., Goldin, P. R., Carmona, P. E., & McQuaid, J. R. (2004). The effects of mindfulness meditation on cognitive processes and affect in patients with past depression. *Cognitive therapy and research*, 28(4), 433-455.

[4] Miller, J. J., Fletcher, K., & Kabat-Zinn, J. (1995). Three-year follow-up and clinical implications of a mindfulness meditation-based stress reduction intervention in the treatment of anxiety disorders. *General hospital psychiatry*, 17(3), 192-200.

control, and so they don't have to go through the discomfort and effort of changing a lifestyle that isn't working for them.

Our discomfort zones are where personal transformations happen. Without discomfort, you don't have anything to motivate you to change. You don't have a reason to get any better. It becomes easy to stay where you are instead of reaching for the greatness you are capable of. With discomfort comes growth. Discomfort brings you closer to a life that actually aligns with what and who you truly are.

There are more examples in nature of this principle—examples teaching us how to learn and grow beyond these comfort zones created by the environments and beliefs we live in. Take the story of the salmon. Salmon hatch upstream, in slow, quiet parts of rivers. As they get older and grow bigger, they swim downstream to the ocean, traveling up to 1000 miles to reach the coast, kind of like I did. I grew up in small town, and as I grew and learned, I moved and changed, and now I have lived all over the world. Finally, when the salmon are ready to reproduce, they swim all the way back upstream, against the tide, over huge rocks, and up waterfalls and past a lot of fishermen.

When the salmon come to a cascade, they jump over it. If the jump fails, they swim around a bit to restore their energy, then try to jump over the cascade again. If they fail, they keep trying until they succeed. They avoid fisherman, bears, and other wildlife that enjoy eating them. The salmon fight and fight to make their way back to the stream where they were hatched, where they lay their eggs. Then, the cycle starts all over again.

What a wonderful life lesson. How comfortable do you think that is for the salmon? In the face of endless obstacles and pushing against forces in nature so strong and seemingly uncomfortable, the salmon never gives up its mission. The salmon knows its natural life cycle involves this journey home through what seems to be a lot of discomfort and pain. The salmon knows it must overcome these trials to fulfill its purpose and takes on the challenges and obstacles with every ounce of strength and energy it has.

This again brings to light the importance of perception. I doubt the mind of the salmon is filled with fear, negativity, frustrations, drugs, or counseling. In fact, they may even enjoy the challenges, making the entire journey a really great experience. Possibly that's why they keep doing it generation after generation. How can you be like a salmon and begin to enjoy your journey?

Our bodies have a similar innate wisdom in relationship to our natural life cycle. Discomfort and pain are an indicator to move, explore, and fight for what we believe is important to our own personal journeys. Just like the salmon, we must overcome hardships to get to where we're truly meant to be, to fulfill our life's purpose. What's amazing about being human is that we also have a natural desire to thrive and feel good. We want to be happy and feel fulfilled, so achieving and maintaining it is even easier when we become aware of it all. Modern medicine and a "normal" lifestyle filled with technology and exciting spectacles to keep us amused and busy in our free time has made it very easy to stay in survival mode, or even totally numb mode. But, you deserve more than just surviving, dealing with it, and learning to live with it. You deserve extraordinary. That's why I'm passionate about the tools and keys I believe will support you in living an extraordinary life.

The stories of the lobster and the salmon show us that discomfort is a signal to tune in and discover where we can grow next. It may not be the easy road, but it's the road we need to take, and will be grateful we did. Discomfort should motivate us to look at and make very serious choices about our environments, the people we are sharing our time with, the work and hobbies we put our time and energy into, the food and products we are choosing to put in and on our bodies, and so on. All of these choices directly determine how we experience this journey we are on, and the kind of body we do it in. From this place, you can create the path to help you get out of survival mode and get into thriving. You'll find that you will enjoy exceptional levels of success in all areas of your life as you grow outside of your comfort zone and live an extraordinary life.

Find Comfort in Discomfort

If you want to live a truly extraordinary life, you cannot look for ways to escape every discomfort. I believe if you really want to achieve, to be the best version of yourself, and to live the life you want, then you must be use and take control of your discomfort. You must set goals and make wise choices to encourage your true magnificence to shine. You have to make the *choice* to embrace your discomfort and learn from it, instead of finding ways to avoid it. You have to stop taking pills or substances that simply help you ignore that unease. To become extraordinary, you have to embrace your discomfort, then learn how to use it to drive yourself forward.

Please, don't let anything or anyone stop you. Avoid the negative people who want to keep you down and away from that exceptional you. Don't give your power away, forget your dreams, and ignore the life you can clearly imagine living. Never allow your friends, foes, family, doctors, media, or anything else support you in staying where you know you really don't want to be, doing what you don't want to be doing, and living a life you no longer are enjoying. Don't allow your fear of change, or the fear of upsetting someone else, keep you in a life where you are unfulfilled, unhappy, anxious, depressed, or sick. You deserve to live a happy, healthy, extraordinary life, and you have the power to choose to live it.

Take this moment and realize you have the power and the ability to make a change, right here and right now. This is a moment when you can embrace where you are in discomfort as your body's natural signal. That signal is telling you to look at your life and find what can you do differently so you can become the healthier, happier, stronger, more successful natural you.

This is a pivotal moment for you. "This is not a dress rehearsal." You can make the choice to act on your discomfort. You can choose to make the hard decisions, to molt your hard outer shell so you can grow. You can choose to swim upstream so you can fulfill the greater purpose that your life is mean to have. What choice will you make?

Key Takeaways:

Your body, mind, emotions, and attitude are all highly affected by whatever you habitually choose to put in, on, and around your body.

Discomfort might be the body's way of telling us that we need to look at what is going on in our minds and lives. You can't escape all discomfort, but you can use it to empower yourself.

If you want to live the life you love and love the life you live, you need to embrace the discomfort in your life. You need to learn from that discomfort and discover how that discomfort can make you a better, happier, healthier, and more successful person.

YOU are in control of the decisions you make about all aspects of your life, especially your health and well-being. You have the power of choice, and the intelligence to educate yourself so you are clear on what the right choices are for you.

Beliefs—Are they supporting your success, or are they ensuring your failure? Are you fighting for your limitations and spending your time, money, and energy on supporting a life of 'issues'? Or, are you allowing your awareness to gently guide you to a life of happiness and empowerment?

Remember, if you have children, what you are teach them will drastically impact their future, and ensure they are happy, healthy, fulfilled, empowered, and successful . . . or not.

"

In life, you need many
more things besides
talent. Things like
good advice
and common sense.

—HACK WILSON

What Advice Should You Follow?

O verall happiness, health, and well-being should be your number-one priority because without it, you won't feel good, have amazing energy, get enthusiastic for life, or achieve high levels of success. It's pointless to get fanatical about weight loss or making your first million dollars if it results in stress, eating disorders, loss of self-esteem and confidence, or ill health or losing who you really are while forgetting what you really want. But how should you get healthy, and how can you maintain your health?

If you're like most people, you're probably overwhelmed when thinking about how to move forward with your health, heal your body, find happiness, or reach a level of success you could have never imagined for yourself. Chances are, you've probably tried a few things that haven't worked. Most attempts to achieve and maintain high levels of health, happiness, and success end up with disappointment, and usually that's because you follow the wrong people and plans. I am always surprised by the amount of bad information shared and spewed on social media. It's no wonder why there is so much frustration and so many failed dreams.

There is also a *lot* of conflicting advice out there. That's why I want to help you identify the advice that is harmful to you so that you can make better choices. There's no point in wasting time and money on gimmicks that not only do not help you improve your life but can also be harmful to you. In this chapter, I'll walk you through an overview of the biggest issues people face when it comes to health, with some advice from traditional medicine as it relates to prescription drugs.

How do you figure out what advice you should follow? In addition to the world of conflicting, bad-vs.-good advice and information you see every day in the media, you also have a world inside of you filled with conflicting information. The lifestyle I promote will guide and support you to eliminate all of the noise and really tune in to what it is you truly need to be the best version of you.

Is Your Mentor Getting Results?

I strongly believe in the value of working with the right mentor for the right reasons. The right mentor for you will save you time, money, confusion and frustration. He or she will have the ability to take you further then you thought possible, while knowing how to guide and support you to actually achieve your goals, rather than just telling you that with the right attitude or information you can achieve 'whatever.'

As stated by two of my clients:

"Retaining Reginald was the best thing I ever did; the cost of his service was earned back 100,000-fold. The consequences of trying to save a buck and not investing in myself is devastating not only to every aspect of my life but also to my family's life."

*"Dear Mr. Reg Lenney—The Holistic Coach. I have just completed my first month of your Holistic Health Program and all I can say is WOW!! You did explain what I could expect. I did read many of your testimonials, but nothing prepared me for your work, your professionalism and the results. **I am speechless!***

"All I can say is everyone needs to try your programs. Anyone who is tired of living with pain and weight problems. *Anyone who is tired of doctors feeding you pills and **telling you to 'learn to live with it.'** Anyone who is not living their life to the fullest. Anyone who is telling themselves that "this is the way I am and I'm ok with it . . ."* This is the best thing you could ever do for yourself! I promise you, Reg Lenney is the real thing and you will thank yourself for taking this step towards living the life you have always wanted, in the body you have always wanted.*

"Thank you again and again!! God bless you."

You won't get the results you want when you fail to get the right advice and information to actually achieve the results you want, with the best tried, tested, and proven strategies and techniques available, set out in the right ways, to fit your individuality and lifestyle. How long have you been trying to maintain high levels of health, happiness, and success, but for some reason you still feel like you just can't quite get where you want to be? Whose advice or guidance have you been trusting?

> It may be wise to learn from others' mistakes, but when you learn from others' success, you will truly fly.

What makes advice *bad* advice? Bad advice comes from people who are not clear about what you really need and why. Our world today is full of "specialists" and "experts." Social media and the internet are packed with advice from "specialists" and those with the good intention to help. But, they never deal with what the real issue is: it's never just one thing, everything affects everything, and you and your lifestyle are unique. Generally, avoid comments, articles, and fad programs that claim that if a strategy is good for one person, it's good for you, too.

It's extremely important to get advice from someone who truly lives what they teach and has the experience of working directly with many, many different types of people. Even those who claim they specifically specialize in one particular type of individual with one specific type of goal, are not able to fully and often times correctly guide you through your particular issues if they do not get fully involved with who you are, with the beliefs you have, in the lifestyle you are living. You can't always trust you'll get the results you want because you can see someone else doing it. I get positive feedback from the individuals I have had the opportunity to help because they see I am committed to living this lifestyle in every aspect of my own life. And, I get fully involved to clearly understand their lives so I can guide them through the right steps to the find awareness that they need. It feels great to be recognized as a mentor and coach who is willing to do the work *with* you.

It always concerns me when I walk into a gym and see someone working with a personal trainer who looks like they have never exercised in their life. Often times, that trainer is not paying attention to how the client is doing the exercise. They ignore what the right exercises are for the individual living the lifestyle they are living in the body they are now living it in.

> ## Taking a few weeks or months' worth of courses or basic training and hanging a few certifications on the wall does not make anyone an expert, despite having gone through three or four bad marriages, bad health issues, and failed businesses.

These days, there are so many unhappy, unprofessional, overweight, out-of-shape, and highly stressed-out mentors, coaches, counselors, trainers, gurus, and specialists, dealing with their own endless personal unresolved issues and incomplete and inaccurate training. It's no wonder why most people are not achieving the results they wish for and are paying for.

It's common to see advertising for courses and programs for almost anyone to become some sort of "specialist" in just a short period of time. In fact, just now I did a Google search for "become a coach" and 136 *million* results came up. I have personal experience working with many, many different types of "specialists" from around the world, as well as experience with many organizations and associations. Many of them use sales and marketing wording as professional fact, such as "[the organization or association] is committed to maintaining and promoting excellence in coaching. Therefore, [it] expects all members and credentialed coaches (coaches, coach mentors, coaching supervisors, coach trainers or students), to adhere to the elements and principles of *ethical* conduct." Wow, that sounds great. However, after many years of personal and very extreme experience with the management, members, and experts from a few of these associations, the facts are very different then the marketing and sales statements they use. It seems that the actual goal of these type of organization is to have as many members as possible paying regular fees, rather than actually ensuring that everyone representing such titles, and in the powerful and influential position to hold the title, is in fact able and capable of being in that position.

Taking a few weeks or months' worth of courses or basic training and hanging a few certifications on the wall does not make anyone an expert, despite having gone through three or four bad marriages, bad health issues, and failed businesses. Anyone putting themselves out there as a "specialist" to help others with anything must have more than just "adequate training." It is also vital for a coach to have personal experience of how to navigate through the challenges and hurdles the client is going to go through, so as to effectively support them through it. It may be wise to learn from others mistakes, but when you learn from others success, you will truly fly.

If you want to improve your life in any way, and you're searching for or open to advice to incorporate into your own life, make sure the person or people you pay your good money to, and trust your life with, are at least already achieving what you want to achieve and more. They should be in their position because they truly want and can help you, instead of being focused on earning a living. And avoid all those free or introductory sessions with trainees who want to test their skills out on you while trying to figure it all out, unless you have a lot of extra time and you are already fully successful in the area they are training in, so you can protect yourself.

Conflicting Advice

It is clearly obvious to me WHY there is so much contradictory and conflicting information, advice, and opinions out there. Rather than them all being "wrong," it may, in fact, actually be that they all work, but for certain people in specific situations.

Only one thing is worse than the sheer *quantity* of information available today on diet, lifestyle, and success: the fact that so much of that information is coming from people who want to sell you yet another magic pill, potion, or "secret strategy." Almost all of the information I read is contradictory, incomplete, and just plain wrong, not to mention the fact that it may not fit your lifestyle or body type. Even industry professionals such as registered dietitians, research scientists, MDs, PhDs, and certified personal trainers give completely contradictory advice. There are a lot of opinions out there, and everyone seems to tell you something different. Most experts can't agree on what remedies, diets, fads, prescriptions, and/or exercise programs work best, and this reinforces my point and message. *There is no one-size-fits-all plan or program that actually gets you complete results long term.*

> ## It is clearly obvious to me WHY there is so much contradictory and conflicting information, advice, and opinions out there.

How do you bypass the marketing lies of the big health or weight loss corporations? How do you cut through the information jungle? How do you sort through the conflicting opinions? When you're diagnosed with something, how do you avoid the fear and pressure to do "whatever" forced on you by the "specialists" and your family and friends? You've already found the solution—and you're reading it. I invite you to follow the common-sense, real-life techniques found here in this book and I promise you, not only will you lose unwanted body fat, but your whole life will become better as you become happier and healthier. Plus, you will have a lot of extra cash in your pocket from avoiding all of the scams, bad information, and endless supply of pills and potions. Buying into the fads, quick-fix guarantees, magic pills, and potions and the belief that "nothing can be done" and "you must learn to live with it" will only lead you down a path to disappointment and a less-than-satisfactory life.

Unlearning the Misinformation You've Learned

Instead of teaching you about fat loss lies, myths, and deceptions, I could have easily dived right into the how-to and mechanics of eating and training for fat loss. However, because of the amount of misinformation in the health and fitness industry today, my job as the author and educator has become very difficult. Before I can effectively begin to teach you the truth about getting healthier, leaner, more muscular, happier, and more successful, I first have to *unteach*, or at least help you to become aware of, the beliefs, rumors, myths, and lies.

The first myth you must un-learn is that your beliefs, choices, environment, habits, lifestyle and the products you use have no effect on your health, happiness, success, and performance. The truth is, your home and work environment, the cleaning products you use, and the bed you sleep in . . . all the way up to the laundry detergents, toothpaste, and antiperspirants you use absolutely do contribute to the unsatisfactory results, pain, stress, weight gain, bad relationships and home life, unfulfilling job, failures, and sluggishness you may be experiencing or dealing with.

The second—and perhaps biggest—myth is that you can follow a one-size-fits-all approach and see long-term results. You're told that if you're a 50-year-old working a corporate desk job, you'll see the same results if you just eat like a 25-year-old who has time to spend hours at the gym every day. I think you know from experience that this isn't true. The people who are successful with these fad programs and diets live a very different lifestyle than you do. To successfully get healthy, increase your energy, achieve your goals, lose weight, and start living the life you love and loving the life you live long term, you must create the right program for *your* lifestyle, personality type, and body type.

Misinformation and the Weight Loss Industry

If all of the weight loss plans, programs, and pills out in the marketplace actually worked, people wouldn't still be buying them. People wouldn't need the next new fad because they'd already have the solution to their weight loss problems. The truth is, no matter how many before-and-after photos a fitness, weight loss, or success program shows in its advertising, there are no quick fixes. There's no magic program or pill that's going to make your fat melt off in a few weeks and help you keep it off long term. You have to forget that bad advice and misinformation if you really want to achieve your health and lifestyle goals, and maintain them.

So how do you know what advice to follow? How do you cut through the misinformation to find plans or programs that actually work for you? Here are a few important tips for navigating the world of weight loss:

- Crash diets don't work and they are not gratifying in the long run. They can even be dangerous.

- Most weight-loss programs are not long-term life plans and fail to resolve and address the real issues that are making you gain weight, like your relationships, environment, or beliefs.

- Calorie-controlled weight loss systems and those crazy programs that tell you to cut something out completely from your diet are doomed to long-term failure. That is, unless you're told to cut out sugar and processed foods completely—that actually works for everyone. You may lose weight at first, but you'll eventually wind up putting on more weight. These programs slow down your metabolism and mess with your leptin levels, making you burn even fewer calories than you did before, and they often make you gain even more weight as a result.

- Most supplements you buy are nothing more than disguised sugar products. Sugar is actually a sedative drug, which has no nutritional or health value whatsoever.

- Intense exercise, either for a weekend or week-long "boot camp," will do little to help you control your weight long term. It may actually be entirely counterproductive to both your health and your fitness, and may often be quite harsh and unenjoyable, not to mention the long-term injuries or damage usually caused by these programs.

- Health and fitness are not the same. You can be fit but not healthy, or, you can be healthy but not fit.

- Following the wrong physical exercise regime can create long-term injury, pain, and energy loss. It can also age your body much faster than normal.

Blindly following what everyone else does when they go to the gym can result in less-than-ideal or even disastrous results. Reading the latest fitness magazine or following along with the newest health blog is not the answer.

As we discussed earlier, you are unique and so is your life, your routine, your body, and your needs. If you have a desk job and you expect that doing two hours in the gym, three times a week and eating the newest health product is going to get you that beach body promoted on the cover of this month's health magazine, and make you "healthy," you will be very disappointed.

> You have to forget that bad advice and misinformation if you really want to achieve your health and lifestyle goals, and maintain them.

Why Fad Diets, Lifestyles and Pills Don't Work

Fad diets, lifestyles, and pills usually limit essential macronutrients, which are fats, proteins, and carbohydrates, as well as micronutrients like vitamins and minerals. Proteins build our muscles and the nutrients in fat help our heart stay healthy. Carbohydrates provide us with energy. Additionally, we need the right balance of vitamins and minerals for our bodies to function normally. An imbalance or insufficiency will affect your mental alertness and resistance to infections, as well as many other vital processes in your body. Vitamins and minerals also enable your body to process the nutrients you eat. Certain vitamins help you produce healthy blood cells, hormones, genetic material, and chemicals in your nervous system. These nutrients are needed and required for a healthy, well-balanced diet.

If you want to lose body fat and keep it off, it's vital to pay attention to how and when you are fueling your machine, your body, as well as how much water you are drinking daily. It's also vital that you have a nutritional intake that contains the right balance of the right fuel that you as an individual require to match your body type, lifestyle, activity levels, and goals. While they can occasionally be supplemented, it's best to get everything your body needs from whole food ingredients and natural additions. The more natural your lifestyle and diet, the more naturally your body performs. Your body is designed to consume *natural* food, not processed pseudo-food.

But again, this is only one more small part of the big picture. Nutrition itself is only one part of the whole. If you only focus on your nutrition, you are missing what will create your weight loss success. Ultimately, you need the right intake *plus* the right kind of mindset, habits, lifestyle, activities, and environment. Remember what you've learned from the previous chapters—your mindset and beliefs ultimately control everything.

Many trendy diets and fitness programs compel you to expend great effort both in your diet and amounts of exercise. The problem is, if the diet is not right for you—by that I mean your fuel intake must match your lifestyle—then you are wasting your time and money, and most likely setting yourself up for injuries and illness.

Don't Follow a One-Size-Fits-All Approach

Let me share a real-life experience I have had with countless clients, and myself. Let's say you have a job or lifestyle that has you stationary most of the time. Maybe you're a corporate executive, an office worker, a truck driver, or you're in some other role that has you sitting or sedentary for hours and hours every day. Many of you are not moving for 15–22 hours a day on average, including working, sleeping and relaxing. Just think for a minute on how actively you actually are making your body move on a daily basis. I'm not talking about just moving your eyes and fingers.

I have never been a person to work in an office or behind a desk regularly, but it became very obvious to me when I started writing books and programs just how fast the entire day can fly by. I have to admit that there were more than a few days that I woke up in the morning, grabbed my computer with the thoughts of just working for just a few minutes, before breakfast or exercise, to ensure I wrote out my thoughts. But, I quickly realized that the entire day was gone, the sun was setting and I hadn't moved, except a quick toilet break or to grab a little snack. I surprised myself with how I could actually work non-stop with no proper food, no water, and almost no breaks, just full on with the computer. I know people who do this almost every day, for years! Be aware of how much you're moving, and how much you're not.

What if your new intention is to achieve that great beach body for summer? The next time you are at the grocery store, you buy the latest fitness magazine, or you go online to see how your favorite actor or actress achieves their great movie-star body. You research fitness programs for stars like Halle Berry from *Catwoman*, Gerard Butler from *300*, or Hugh Jackman from *X-Men*, three clients I have been blessed to work with. Let's say you start following the latest celebrity nutrition and fitness program. The program has you eat five or more healthy meals a day and squeeze in time at the gym three, four, or maybe even six times a week, depending on your goals.

Let me be brutally honest with you. The chances of you achieving the results promised by the 'celebrity plan' are slim to none, given your work and lifestyle. Your body isn't ready for or able to do this, nor will your lifestyle support it. And here is an 'insiders secret' from working with endless movie stars, models, and even professional athletes: most of the time those people don't even look like their pictures in real life. And, if you hear any interviews they have done regarding the roles they played, they state that maintaining those awesome bodies is nearly impossible after the shoot, and these guys have all the money and support to do it.

> Health and fitness are not the same. You can be fit but not healthy, or, you can be healthy but not fit.

The next problem with this kind of program is that even when you do achieve a small amount of success, it is often too difficult to maintain for long periods of time. This is why so many people spend endless amounts of time, money, and energy yo-yo dieting as a normal part of their lives. You completely alter your lifestyle for a week or two, or even a few months, only to find that your new lifestyle doesn't actually work for your life, or you just can't wait to get back to your former routine. So, you go back to your old, unhealthy habits, gaining back the weight you lost—and then some.

What about the liquid diet for a week program? Liquid cleanses, juice cleanses, and detox programs are gaining a lot of attention in the media, and they are big business. Of course, you will lose weight, but you will most likely gain it back the following week when you go back to your "normal" life. Why not forget the extremes and incorporate juicing in a fun and maintainable way into your life so as to enjoy the benefits all year round? When you move too far to one extreme, the pendulum will always swing back the other way. The problem is that these fad diets are not sustainable, and they won't provide your body what it needs to be nourished, creating imbalances rather than great health.

What about people you know or see that do look great all year round? The reality is, these actors, professional athletes, fitness magazine models (and most of the people you see on the beach with great bodies) live very different lives than you do. I don't care what program you follow, what magic pills and potions you're taking, or how many times you go to the gym. These people look amazing because they live that way all day every day. They eat the right foods and spend hours in the gym every day. They get to bed by 10 or 11 every night and get a full night's sleep. Then, they get up early and hit the gym again. They also incorporate yoga classes, regular massage therapy sessions, all the right supplements, and they generally have the time and money to relax and enjoy a stress-free life with people they want to be with. Their full-time job is to look the way they do. So how are you going to achieve what they do in a fraction of the time, with a very different lifestyle?

What Works for Weight Loss

If you want to achieve your perfect weight, a healthy and powerful body, have a clear and powerful mind, and maintain high levels of natural energy, you must learn to live happily, have fun, and be healthy every day. It must become a lifestyle, not a temporary trial where you endlessly bounce from one program to another and one diet to another. You have to find a program that you can sustain long term, a program teaching you a lifestyle that removes the stress and frustration. You need a set of customized strategies and techniques that are easy to implement and fun to incorporate, strategies that enhance and excite you and that consistently provide you with the results you want long term. What you don't need is another program to follow for a few weeks and then quickly forget about.

Metabolism is a biological process that your body utilizes to convert food into energy. If you're the average person, your metabolism adapts itself to your body's daily needs. The foods you're eating, when and how much you eat, your sleep habits, your activity levels, your stress levels, and the condition of your body, and of course your environment, all affect your metabolism. If you're inactive—maybe you're a couch potato, or maybe you just spend hours at a computer every day—your metabolism will be slow. If you are athletic or very active, you will have much more energy during the day.

People with more muscle tone burn more calories per day than a person who has more body fat. Your body needs physical activity to create more energy and increase your metabolic rate. Like the old saying goes, "If you don't use it, you lose it." If you sit around all day, why would your body bother to burn high levels of calories to make energy you don't need? Your body works very efficiently, so if you don't need a lot of energy to fuel activity, your body won't create it. Your metabolism slows down, and your body stores more of the calories you eat as fat. Conversely, the more physically active you are, the more lean muscle you will have, and the more calories you burn, even while you're sleeping. That is why being active is so vital to weight-loss.

> If you want to achieve your perfect weight, a healthy and powerful body, have a clear and powerful mind, and maintain high levels of natural energy, you must learn to live happily, have fun, and be healthy every day.

Nutrition programs with overly low-calorie diets are not healthy or sustainable. If you don't eat enough, your body will go into a starvation mode to protect itself. Drastically limiting your calories will actually slow down your metabolism, making your body store even more fat. That's why very low-calorie diets are actually counterproductive. Unless you are under the supervision of a doctor, never use a diet with less than 1000 calories per day. The body needs the energy to circulate blood, walk, breathe, and even think. If it is starved of necessary calories, it will go into a conservation mode and burn fewer calories, and you won't lose any fat.

What about taking a pill for weight loss? Diet pills interfere with our natural body functions. They disturb the balance of hormones, causing you to become addicted to the pills. Many of these pills also have detrimental side effects, doing more harm than good. There is no magic pill to lose weight, and they haven't invented a "happy pill" that won't eventually make you very unhappy.

Medications Can Be Dangerous

Like weight loss, there's also a lot of misinformation out there about the pharmaceutical industry and medications. In fact, even more than diet and weight loss, my clients and most people I speak with have many false beliefs about drugs and pharmaceuticals, based on misinformation, misunderstandings, and false "facts." The next section of the book will explore different areas related to the dangers of prescription and over-the-counter drugs and why fad pills and diets don't work.

Are you aware of what prescription drugs are doing to you and your family? They can be just as dangerous as the illegal ones, often even more so. And, of course, they're much easier to get hold of. More people die every year from doctor-prescribed legal drugs than any other cause. How many celebrities have we lost in our lifetimes because they overdosed on legal pharmaceuticals? And, why are common over-the-counter and prescription drugs so dangerous? Let's dive in to the hazards of the pills that are common, and normal, to regularly take.

> We oftentimes don't realize the dangers of floating through life in 'automatic mode,' just doing what everyone else does or says, just because everyone else is saying and doing it.

We view medicines as safe because they are manufactured in a medical lab setting, accepted by society as helpful, sanctioned by the government through the Federal Drug Administration, and offered to us by "specialists" who are regulated by a licensing organization. We oftentimes don't realize the dangers of floating through life in 'automatic mode,' just doing what everyone else does or says, just because everyone else is saying and doing it. Abusing prescription drugs, because we are less familiar with the long-term effects of taking them, has completely and totally changed our world. Also, many of us have no frame of reference since many of these types of drugs didn't exist in our youth.

Yes, people have benefited from today's prescription drugs. After all, we are told they are supposed to be designed to help us heal, manage illness, prolong life, or provide much-needed comfort. They are often used to improve the quality of our lives, and in many cases, they do. So, what's the problem?

The problem is that when medicines are misused or abused, they come with risks and dangers equivalent to or worse than any issue the patient may have had in the first place. And, due to the normality of it all, they tend to cause much deeper and longing-lasting issues than those of using street drugs. They can lead to dependence and addiction with the same consequences (or more) as those of heroin or any other street drug. Remember how we spoke about sugar being up to eight times more addictive to heroin, and all the problems that it brings? Big business is about making big money, so to keep you coming back, you must really want to. There's no clearer example of this than the current prescription opioid overdose epidemic occurring in America. Abuse of legal, prescribed medicines is even more lethal than illegal street drugs, as we regularly witness on the news and in social media.

How do I know that prescription drugs are so dangerous? For over 32 years, I have been working with clients suffering from drug dependency, depression, weight problems, stomach problems, liver problems, skin problems, memory problems, digestive problems, family problems, work problems, and life problems that all stem from the use of prescription drugs. I have seen people do terrible things that they would have never done if not for these "safe" drugs. I consistently work with children who are nowhere near "normal," already taking handfuls of pharmaceuticals and clearly set up for an entire lifetime of more. I have seen and heard of countless more being involved in violent crimes as a result of prescription drug use, and many of these medications are known catalysts for suicide.

In fact, individuals suffering from depression are many hundreds of times more likely to commit a crime[1] or suicide[2] while on doctor-prescribed, legal pharmaceuticals than those who are not on any sort of prescription medication at all. Please always be aware of all medicines and products you choose to bring into your home. Research them, understand them, and know what they are doing to you and your family. If you do choose to take anything, always control it and set a clear timeline for how long you are going to use it, only as a temporary support while you are working to control and 'fix' your health.

---

[1] Molero, Y., Lichtenstein, P., Zetterqvist, J., Gumpert, C. H., & Fazel, S. (2015). Selective serotonin reuptake inhibitors and violent crime: a cohort study. *PLoS medicine*, 12(9), e1001875.

[2] Gibbons, R. D., Brown, C. H., Hur, K., Marcus, S. M., Bhaumik, D. K., Erkens, J. A., ... & Mann, J. J. (2007). Early evidence on the effects of regulators' suicidality warnings on SSRI prescriptions and suicide in children and adolescents. *American journal of psychiatry*, 164(9), 1356-1363.

Here are some facts about prescription drug misuse and abuse taken from The Institute for Safe Medication Practices (ISMP)[3]:

• Every day, 2,500 teenagers use a prescription drug to get high for the first time.

• Twelve- to seventeen-year-olds abuse prescription drugs more than they abuse ecstasy, crack/cocaine, heroin, and methamphetamine combined.

• The number of new abusers of prescription drugs is now greater than the number of brand new users of marijuana, according to the Substance Abuse and Mental Health Services Administration.

• Abuse of prescription painkillers causes more deaths than heroin and cocaine combined, according to the Drug Enforcement Administration.

> If you do choose to take anything, always control it and set a clear timeline for how long you are going to use it, only as a temporary support while you are working to control and 'fix' your health.

A Prescription for Problems

I've spent a lot of time researching the dangers of prescription medications. Through that research, I compiled a list of the worst prescription drug offenders, medications that cause people to become violent towards others and themselves. Among the top-ten most dangerous are the antidepressants Pristiq (desvenlafaxine), Paxil (paroxetine), and Prozac (fluoxetine). These medications were created to help eliminate depression, yet they've been shown to make it up to 800% more likely that a person will commit suicide on the drug than if they had never taken it.

Concerns about the extremely negative effects of many popular antidepressants and antipsychotic drugs have been on the rise, as these

---

[3] Institute for Safe Medication Practices. (2017). Retrieved July 11, 2017 from http://www.ismp.org.

drugs not only cause severe health problems to users, but also pose a significant threat to society. The ISMP report indicates that many popular prescription drugs are linked even to homicides. So, these medications not only affect those who take them, but also the people around them.

Most of the top ten most dangerous drugs are antidepressants, but the list also includes insomnia medication (think of Michael Jackson), attention-deficit hyperactivity disorder (ADHD) drugs (remember my story of the mom with three kids), a malaria drug, and anti-smoking medication.[4] Here is the full list:

1. **Desvenlafaxine** (Pristiq)—Antidepressant that affects serotonin and noradrenaline. The drug is 7.9 times more likely to be associated with violence than other drugs.

2. **Venlafaxine** (Effexor)—Antidepressant that treats anxiety disorders. The drug is 8.3 times more likely to be associated with violence than other drugs.

3. **Fluvoxamine** (Luvox)—A selective serotonin reuptake inhibitor (SSRI) drug that is 8.4 times more likely to be associated with violence than other drugs.

4. **Triazolam** (Halcion)—A benzodiazepine drug for insomnia that is 8.7 times more likely to be associated with violence than other drugs.

5. **Atomoxetine** (Strattera)—An ADHD drug that is 9 times more likely to be associated with violence than other drugs.

6. **Mefoquine** (Lariam)—A malaria drug that is 9.5 times more likely to be associated with violent behavior than other drugs.

7. **Amphetamines**—This general class of ADHD drug is 9.6 times more likely to be associated with violence than other drugs.

---

[4] Szalavitz, M. (2011). Top Ten Legal Drugs Linked to Violence. Retrieved July 11, 2017 from http://healthland.time.com/2011/01/07/top-ten-legal-drugs-linked-to-violence/.

8. **Paroxetine** (Paxil)—A SSRI antidepressant drug that is 10.3 times more likely to be associated with violence than other drugs. It is also linked to severe withdrawal symptoms and birth defects.

9. **Fluoxetine** (Prozac)—A popular SSRI antidepressant drug that is 10.9 times more likely to be associated with violence than other drugs.

10. **Varenicline** (Chantix)—An anti-smoking drug that is a shocking 18 times more likely to be associated with violence than other drugs.

All of these drugs are regularly and freely given to millions of people every day by "specialists" who are supposed to be looking after the best interest of their clients. Before subjecting yourself or a loved one to any of these types of medications, please do take the time to educate yourself. Make sure you understand the consequences of taking these medications so you can make an informed decision whether you should actually subject yourself or anyone else to taking them.

> Make sure you understand the consequences of taking these medications so you can make an informed decision whether you should actually subject yourself or anyone else to taking them.

I also strongly encourage you to try the easy-to-implement methods outlined in this book. These are methods that have proven success and no negative side effects at all. Choose to take an honest look at yourself, your life, and your choices. Choose to resolve your issues before settling for something that you are told will help you live with your issues, but that in reality will only cause many more. You'll find that in most cases, you don't even need these medications in the first place. And, if you actually do need some sort of pharmaceutical, plan to use them as a support to correcting the issue, and use them temporarily, for as short of period of time possible, rather than living a lifestyle where pharmaceuticals are a normal and regular part of your life.

Aspirin: A Loaded Gun for Your Heart

Over-the-counter drugs aren't always safe. Take aspirin for example. Should you use aspirin to help your heart? The drug companies want you to think of aspirin as a magic bullet for your heart. Many doctors recommend low-dose aspirin to their patients who are at an increased risk of getting heart disease or having a heart attack. Oh, it's a bullet all right—and it's aimed at your ticker.

There are many, many downright crazy beliefs about pharmaceuticals. One of the most irritatingly persistent myths in modern medicine is the downright insane notion that daily aspirin can help your heart. I can't tell you how it lifts my own heart to see this falsehood finally crumbling. Even the Wall Street Journal is finally giving aspirin therapy the kiss of death. A recent story with the headline "The Danger of Daily Aspirin" began with this sentence: "If you're taking a daily aspirin for your heart, you may want to reconsider."[5]

Forget "may"—you should definitely reconsider, because taking a daily aspiring was a bad idea the moment Big Pharma's marketing department dreamed it up.

> Please, for your own benefit, don't gobble down daily aspirin, or take any other pharmaceuticals regularly just because a drug is available over the counter, or some "specialist" told you to take it.

One new study in the Journal of the American Medical Association found giving aspirin to people at high risk of heart disease provided no benefit at all, just like the chemotherapy myth for cancer. My favorite part is that study was funded in part by Bayer. You see, Bayer invented aspirin in 1899, so it was funny that they funded research that proved their own product has no benefits. It must've been awkward when it came time to deliver the results of the study. I'll bet they're looking for a refund—and a few researchers' heads.

---

[5] Mathews, A. W. (2010). The Danger of Daily Aspirin. Retrieved July 11, 2017 from *https://www.wsj.com/articles/SB10001424052748704511304575075701363436686*.

However, the truth's the truth—and the truth is, aspirin can cause bleeding in the stomach, intestine, and brain, which can lead to a hemorrhagic stroke. Not only does aspirin not prevent heart attacks, but patients who take daily aspirin (or, who take ibuprofen regularly) actually double their risk of a fatal heart attack.[6]

Furthermore:

- People who take aspirin and other NSAIDs (non-steroidal anti-inflammatory drugs) are more likely to die from severe bleeding in the upper gastrointestinal tract.[7]

- If you take aspirin, you're also at an increased risk of getting a hemorrhagic stroke, where a blood vessel breaks and blood is released into the brain.[8] (Hemorrhagic strokes only make up about 15% of all strokes, but they account for 40% of stroke deaths,[9] so they're very dangerous.).

- Aspirin is also known to cause hearing loss,[10] which can be worsened if you're regularly around loud noises.[11]

- Regular aspirin use can also cause macular degeneration,[12] which can lead to blindness.

---

[6] Fowkes, F. G. R., Price, J. F., Stewart, M. C., Butcher, I., Leng, G. C., Pell, A. C., ... & Murray, G. D. (2010). Aspirin for prevention of cardiovascular events in a general population screened for a low ankle brachial index: a randomized controlled trial. *JAMA*, 303(9), 841-848.

[7] Lanas, A., Perez-Aisa, M. A., Feu, F., Ponce, J., Saperas, E., Santolaria, S., ... & Navarro, J. M. (2005). A nationwide study of mortality associated with hospital admission due to severe gastrointestinal events and those associated with nonsteroidal antiinflammatory drug use. *The American journal of gastroenterology*, 100(8), 1685.

[8] He, J., Whelton, P. K., Vu, B., & Klag, M. J. (1998). Aspirin and risk of hemorrhagic stroke: a meta-analysis of randomized controlled trials. *JAMA*, 280(22), 1930-1935.

[9] National Stroke Association. (2017). Hemorrhagic stroke. Retrieved from http://www.stroke .org/understand-stroke/what-stroke/hemorrhagic-stroke.

[10] Brien, J. A. (1993). Ototoxicity associated with salicylates. *Drug safety*, 9(2), 143-148.

[11] McFadden, D., & Plattsmier, H. S. (1983). Aspirin can potentiate the temporary hearing loss induced by intense sounds. *Hearing research*, 9(3), 295-316.

[12] Liew, G., Mitchell, P., Wong, T. Y., Rochtchina, E., & Wang, J. J. (2013). The association of aspirin use with age-related macular degeneration. *JAMA internal medicine*, 173(4), 258-264.

What's even more surprising? A daily aspirin regimen may not even help protect you from major cardiovascular events like heart attack and stroke,[13] the reason why your doctor told you to take it in the first place. In a 2010 study published in the Journal of the American Medical Association (JAMA) showed that aspirin did not reduce the risk of vascular events like heart attack or stroke caused by a blood clot.[14] It also had no effect on how long the patients in the study lived. If a daily aspirin doesn't do anything for you, and it can cause terrible side effects, why are you still taking it?

> If you really want to pop a pill or take something to protect your body, mind, and heart, while eliminating inflammation and infection and increasing your health, take some organic omega 3-6-9, and pure Vitamin C Crystals mixed in with a real lemon every day.

Despite aspirin's obvious dangers, you can't turn on the TV without seeing a commercial that talks up aspirin therapy for heart patients. An actress in one commercial claims, "My doctor says it's the easiest preventive measure you can take." Easy? Yes. Safe? Heck no. Sounds like you need a new doctor—one who's been reading the medical journals and is serious about your health and well-being, instead of watching aspirin commercials and looking forward to the next gift or trip to a tropical island, courtesy of the pharmaceutical company.

Here's one fact you won't hear in those ads: roughly half of all people who suffer a fatal heart attack took an aspirin that day. I wonder what their final thoughts were. I bet more than a few clutched their chest and cried

---

[13] Nutri-Spec. *Pharmaceutical Mythology: Do Not Take Aspirin as a Blood Thinner.* Retrieved from http://www.nutri-spec.net/articles/PDF/pm-aspirin.pdf

[14] Fowkes, F. G. R., Price, J. F., Stewart, M. C., Butcher, I., Leng, G. C., Pell, A. C., ... & Murray, G. D. (2010). Aspirin for prevention of cardiovascular events in a general population screened for a low ankle brachial index: a randomized controlled trial. *JAMA*, 303(9), 841-848.

out, "But I took an aspirin today!" There is no magic pill to magically keep you from having a heart attack, and that includes aspirin.

Please, for your own benefit, don't gobble down daily aspirin, or take any other pharmaceuticals regularly just because a drug is available over the counter, or some "specialist" told you to take it. There are exciting and fun looking ads all over the place showing you how great it is to take this stuff. You may even hear about millions of people around the world who take that drug daily and they are still alive. But, that doesn't make it safe, or that it's great for you to take.

These are powerful drugs, not candy, even if many people munch on them like Skittles. If you really want to pop a pill or take something to protect your body, mind, and heart, while eliminating inflammation and infection and increasing your health, take some organic omega 3-6-9. Add in 10 drops of pure organic oil of oregano in a bit of water twice daily, and take two tablespoons of pure organic vitamin C powder in a bottle of pure water and a real lemon squeezed into it twice daily. Try this for a month and you'll be pleasantly surprised by how much better you feel.

Doctors and the Healthcare Industry

As you would have probably guessed, the "healthcare" industry is funded by the drug companies, and therefore most natural care is tagged as dangerous or useless to keep the attention on paid-for corporate pharmaceuticals. This makes healthcare more about the profit than the cure. These big companies need to keep earning. They focus on creating pills that you'll need to take for a lifetime instead of finding a cure.

> Oftentimes doctors don't have the time or knowledge to create a plan to fix that root cause, so they take the simpler route: do their job, follow the rules, and write a prescription.

However, the good news is that things are slowly changing and many good doctors who truly care, and who are holding themselves accountable to honor their beliefs and sworn duty by finally taking a stand for the health and benefit of their patients. I personally work with over a hundred outstanding doctors who regularly send their patients to me to help with ailments that are often considered chronic and incurable. Those conditions can be cured, but not with a medicine cabinet full of pills or a system designed to keep them sick.

We should remember that a doctor's entire education is designed, monitored, and guided by the drug companies. A lot of the time they truly don't know any other way, and often won't even discuss alternative medicines with their patients. It's much easier to prescribe a pill to treat a condition than it is to find the root cause. Oftentimes doctors don't have the time or knowledge to create a plan to fix that root cause, so they take the simpler route: do their job, follow the rules, and write a prescription.

> If you put your health in another's hands, you may lose, as is so common these days.

We all need to take control of our own health, really educate ourselves, and understand and listen to our own bodies. Be your own advocate. Don't be afraid to tell your doctors what you want and ask them if there are other, better, natural ways they would be willing to investigate to help you. If they don't help, find someone else who will help you reach your health goals. If you put your health in another's hands, you may lose, as is so common these days. So, if your doctor or "specialist" is not listening to you, or willing to support you through the journey of eliminating ailments and issues, the answer is simple—get a different doctor.

Follow Your Body

Throughout this book, you'll learn the simple little tweaks and adjustments that will make massive improvements to your mind, body, and lifestyle. You'll discover what choices are best for you and what serves your highest health and success. You'll learn how to follow your own advice because you will be intently aware and trust yourself to know what is best for you and your life goals.

You'll also learn how to design the right nutrition and fitness plans for you. You'll learn how to create a program that's right for you—a program that will match your lifestyle—so you can stop wasting your money and start seeing results. When you start to pay attention to your own body and find what works for you, you'll find the true secret to achieving and maintaining your perfect weight, achieving great health, creating high levels of natural energy, and living a happier life.

Key Takeaways

Health isn't just fitness or a diet—it's a balance of what you put in you, on you, and around you, as well as what you believe, what you focus on, and the people you surround yourself with, as well as your activity levels. Your health is the choices you make every minute of every day that fulfill you, create your passion, and help you live the life you love while you achieve the goals you want, and maintain it all long term.

Most people are failing with their health because of two main things:

1. They are giving away control of their health and wellness to others

2. They are following bad advice from "experts" who are not very clear on what they were dealing with before they started dealing with it.

Beware of the connection between the healthcare industry and the pharmaceutical industry—and know that it does not have *your* best interests at heart.

Make sure you are seeing a doctor who is listening to you and truly willing to help you take control of your health. Find a doctor who looks for the underlying causes of your issues instead of just prescribing medication to address symptoms.

You will never be able to sustain a healthy, successful lifestyle from a fad pill or fad diet. A diet is not the answer—lifestyle change and great choices are the answer.

It is vital that you find the right lifestyle *for you*. You need to find the right advice *for you*. You won't achieve great, long-lasting results from blindly following the plans or programs that are right for someone else. You need to create the strategies that work for you and your unique needs and wants.

The
Natural
You
approach

"

Beliefs have the
power to create and
the power to destroy.
Human beings have
the awesome ability to
take any experience
of their lives and
create a meaning that
disempowers them or
one that can literally
save their lives.

—TONY ROBBINS

Healthy Living and Beliefs

You've tried again and again to live a happier and healthier life. You've followed more diets and workout plans than you can remember, but they haven't worked long term. You may see results for a few weeks or months, but ultimately you go back to your old habits and the weight comes back on. You jump from relationship to relationship, friendship to friendship, never finding anything that feels right. Or worse, you stick with ones that feel wrong because you don't know what else to do, you don't believe you could create the life you want yourself, and you think, "it's better than being alone." Your career isn't what you want it to be— you're totally stressed out, and switching jobs or positions hasn't helped.

What can you do to finally get your life on the right path?

My Natural You approach is the solution you've been looking for. It's a framework that you can use to create an individualized plan for happiness and health. This approach has gotten my clients amazing results thanks to the 10 Keys to Ultimate Health, Happiness, and Success that lay the foundation for my methodology. This chapter will give you a glimpse into the approach and its ability to change your life while guiding you through easy-to-implement steps to help you maintain the changes you achieve.

The 10 Keys

So how does the Natural You approach work? We focus on the 10 biggest parts of your life that are responsible for your health, happiness, success, and satisfaction.

THE 10 KEYS THAT ARE FUNDAMENTAL TO THIS METHOD ARE YOUR:
So how does the Natural You approach work? We focus on the 10 biggest parts of your life that are responsible for your health, happiness, success, and fulfillment.

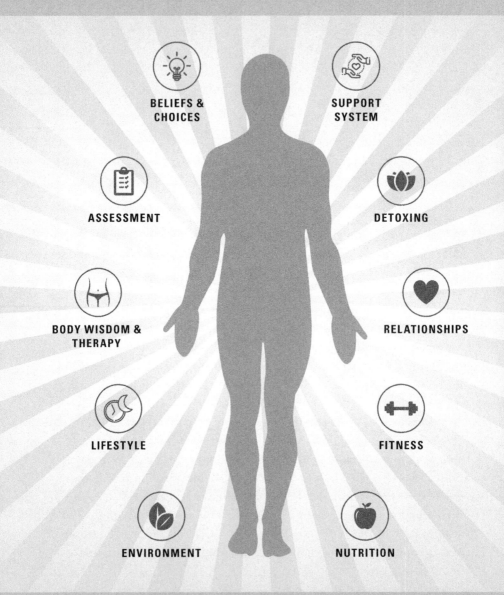

This is the foundation to creating an extraordinary life that you love, in a body you love to live in. Throughout the rest of this book, I'll walk you through how you can use these10 Vital areas and make changes to help you live your happiest, healthiest life.

Can one method really help you and your unique life situation? Yes. I have used these 10 Keys to support clients from all walks of life; from stay at home moms and dads to retirees. I've helped clients going through massive life changes such as relationship troubles, unemployment, addiction, or chronic ailments. And, I've used the same 10 Keys to help top professional athletes, actors, corporate executives, royal families, philanthropists, and very successful business leaders maintain exceptionally high levels of mental and physical performance! These people want to up-level their game and maintain an extraordinary life that gives them access to greater amounts of prosperity, wealth, happiness, and success, and the 10 Keys help them do just that.

> The reality is, no matter who you are, where you came from, where you have been, or where you want to go, your struggles aren't insurmountable.

The reality is, no matter who you are, where you came from, where you have been, or where you want to go, your struggles aren't insurmountable. We are all human beings and we're all dealing with similar core issues that affect how our bodies and minds work, what creates an environment for success, and what holds us back. I am here support you in achieving that powerful, happy, healthy, and successful life that makes you look forward to waking up every morning.

These essential keys are a powerful foundation and have been proven effective over and over in my own life and in the lives of my clients. When you make the choice to take control of your world, I know these keys will enhance all aspects of your life too. This approach *works* because it gets to the root issues that so many other programs ignore, don't fully address, or don't even realize exist. My 10 Keys help you address and overcome these issues so you can move beyond them. When you implement these keys, you'll have the tools to implement the changes you need to live your best life.

Starting with the Natural You Approach

The Natural You approach starts by looking at everything about you and your whole life—your beliefs, environment, body, health, wants and needs, personality, work, family, hobbies, activity levels, pastimes, relationships with food and people, and so on. You determine which areas of life are not working for you with my guidance. Some areas you might be clear about, some you may not be aware of. We start at the foundation of happiness, because if you don't have these keys in place, it doesn't matter if you follow a great workout plan or use the best detox program out there. You won't see long-term results if you don't have that solid foundation.

How will you know if an area of your life is supporting you in your health, happiness, and success or not? Simple: be aware! How do you feel when you think of where you spend your time, something you do daily, or the people you spend your time with? If you think of regular activities or people in your life, what stands out and makes you smile and feel great, and what stands out as bringing down your happiness, passion, and energy? What do you consistently complain about? What are the areas of your life that just don't make you feel good? Your happiness, health, and success must become the priority and be a starting point to move you towards becoming the best version of you.

We have been taught that putting 'you' first is selfish. I believe the total opposite. If you don't put you first, you're not able to be the best 'you' possible. That means you're not able to share the best of who you are with others. How good are you at being a parent, a partner, a creator, or an achiever if you feel like crap? If you are frustrated, have low energy, hate what you're doing or who you're doing it with, how much of 'you' will you actually put into the time spent, and at what level of quality? No matter if you're spending time with your kids or working on a project, you're either going to be magnificent at it, or you will just spend the time working your way through it.

The goal of this practice is to learn to be you, the best you in all areas of your life. You should be the real you, no games, no acting, no trying, no 'working at it.' You should be the real you that makes you enjoy your time. Even when you're doing things you would prefer not doing, you can still find the joy in it if you are working towards your goals and dreams. To get to the core of your failures, fears, ailments, illness, depression, and frustrations, you look at the stress, disappointments, unfulfilling areas, pain, negative patterns, and chronic issues that are preventing you from being the extraordinary person you naturally are, without forcing yourself to 'fit in' to the things that just don't feel right to you. This will become your guidance system for creating a lifestyle you love and that is easy to maintain.

Follow this methodology and you will create a foundation to build upon. You will begin to enjoy high levels of natural energy, and you'll naturally become your perfect weight. Your mind will be so clear, and it will perform so powerfully and efficiently that it will take you to places you never knew could exist. You will be able to maintain peak physical, emotional, and mental performance while you enjoy a connected, strong, loving, intimate, and supportive life. You will learn the ways to achieve victory while avoiding things that take away from your happiness, health, and success.

Getting to the Core

Do you know what the most important element is to you in each of the different areas of your life and/or business? Your beliefs. Your core values and choices are directly related to what you believe in or believe should be. Beliefs shape your perception of the world and why you are exactly where you are in your life, feeling and looking the way you do.

For example, if you believe running will give you the greatest full-body workout that will help you achieve the results you want, then you will choose to run. Here's the catch: you may *believe* running is the best way to achieve the results you want, no matter what, even if you experience aches, pains, or even body damage. You may realize you are destroying your body by running, but you do it anyway. Even if you hate doing it, you will still prioritize running because of your beliefs.

The reality is that you will experience very different feelings and results from running compared to someone who loves it. Those feelings will change the results of your workouts, and everything else you use

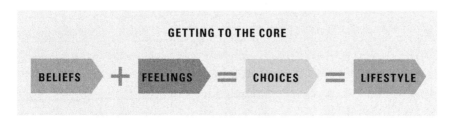

your time and energy for before and after the run. So, the common-sense thing to do would be to either change your beliefs, or change what you're doing.

And, the great thing about beliefs is that you can change them.

That is the funny thing about beliefs—you can believe something will work, but if it does not feel right to you, does not align with what you value, or is something you must force yourself to do because you believe you should, it will ultimately lead to a breakdown in something, somewhere. That belief in a single solution can negatively affect your body, mind, and life. Beliefs are so important because if your beliefs don't align with what you really want in life, you'll never be truly happy or healthy. And, the great thing about beliefs is that you can change them.

What about relationships? Do you believe if you get married, you're married for life? What if, after you get married, you discover the person you married is not the same person you are now living with? What if the person you dedicated your life to changes for the worse? What if, after a few years, you discover you and your partner have very different wants, needs, and goals? What if you wake up in the morning and you don't like the person you're lying next to, and they don't like you, no matter how hard you work at it? When you're driving home after a long day away, do you look forward to getting home, or do you dread it? What if this person you're sharing the best part of yourself with belittles you, abuses you, makes you feel bad about yourself, or crushes your dreams and goals, as I experienced in one of my own relationships, losing my two beautiful daughters in the process.

These are very difficult questions to answer for some people, but they can be some of the most important and powerful questions you've ever asked yourself. If you're not happy with the people you surround yourself with but you believe that you need to stay where you are, you won't ever be happy or fulfilled. That dissatisfaction WILL affect every other part of your life, from your mood at work to your physical health. Your beliefs are ultimately one of the most powerful of the 10 Keys. They affect *everything* in your life, and everything you will ever do and become.

Beliefs, choice, lifestyle, environment and being true to yourself are far more important than any diet, fitness program, detox program, counselor, coach, career, or anything else. If you want to be healthy, powerful, successful, and happy, first make sure that the people and environments you choose to share your life with and give your love, support, and energy to are worthy of it!

I am sharing all of this with you because it is vital that you understand and believe that you have the power and the right to take a close look at the beliefs that aren't working for you in all the different areas of your life. You should also examine the beliefs that don't inspire you to do and be better and feel great. You have the power and the right to choose to make the changes that will support you to be exactly what and how you want to be, long term. Beliefs truly are the core to the entire Natural You approach. That's why I want you to start out by analyzing your beliefs for the next week so you can begin to see and understand what's holding you back.

Your beliefs are ultimately one of the most powerful of the 10 Keys.

I continually educate people about the importance of knowing what you truly believe in. It's important to start by looking at all aspects of your life to achieve great health, happiness, and success. When you focus on the big picture instead of the small details of how to eliminate aches, pains, disease, ailments, and issues from your life, you are laying a foundation for the ultimate YOU. It's important to know the beliefs you've attached to the people, places, and experiences you have in your life. Once you begin to be true to you, once you really become aware, you will be able to determine if your beliefs are serving the best version of you or taking away from it.

When you become aware of your beliefs and the choices you make because of them, it will lead to understanding the choices and lifestyle changes that will support you in letting go of unhealthy habits and behaviors. The key is, notice your environment, make the right choices for you and your lifestyle and make *permanent* changes in your belief systems and daily routines. Get out of the mindset that you are going to 'try this' or 'do that' until you reach a certain goal or to see if it works or not. The goal is to understand the right ways to live for you, then stick with it. Consistency has brought you to where you are right now. If you wish to experience something different, you must consistently make simple little changes, tweaks, and adjustments to ensure you will get to where you truly want to be long term.

Belief is the number one key to changing anything and everything in your life and business. If you are ready to play a bigger game in life, remember to check in with what's most important to you and notice the beliefs that coincide. Notice which ones are yours, and notice which ones were given to you. The power to change your life is in your beliefs. And, the great thing about beliefs are; you can change them.

> **Beliefs, choice, lifestyle, environment and being true to yourself are far more important than any diet, fitness program, detox program, counselor, coach, career, or anything else.**

The *Natural You* Daily Practice

For the next seven days, I invite you to look at ONE area of your life that you have complaints, frustrations, or anxiety around. Answer the following questions:

1. How are your thoughts, feelings, and beliefs affecting your way of being? "Way of being" means how you are feeling and behaving at work, at home, or in your relationships. Perhaps you're living with constant complaints, frustrations, and uneasiness due to different issues you consistently deal with. Are your thoughts, feelings, and beliefs empowering you, igniting your passion, encouraging your goals, and supporting your needs—or are they taking away from your energy, passion, power, and goals?

2. What beliefs are present for you? Are they important to you? If so, why?

3. Why do you hold these beliefs? Is it because of something you read somewhere, because someone told you this is the way it is or it's supposed to be, or because this was the way you were brought up throughout your childhood?

Consider an example of the power of your beliefs. Your doctor recommends cutting sugar out of your diet to benefit your health and mental performance, but you love your indulgence in sugary delights. It will be much more challenging to cut out sugar because you believe your sugary treats are important to you, or necessary in order to have the energy you need to do what needs to be done. You may not even believe it's possible you could be addicted to sugar, or that it is bad for you. When you start, you may not even understand what beliefs are holding you back. That's why you must continue asking yourself the questions listed above over and over until you begin to understand those beliefs.

The Importance of Environment

Your environment affects whether your body and mind are healthy or not. If you are living in an unhealthy environment, you can develop unhealthy beliefs about yourself or the people in it. This kind of thinking will support making unhealthy choices that lead to unhappiness and dis-ease in your body and mind. Toxic environments are too much for the body and mind to maintain, ensuring your goals of great health, happiness, and success will always come last.

Everything around you influences your lifestyle choices. What you believe, how you choose to behave, your work and home environments, your relationships, your levels of physical activity, the foods you choose to eat and how much of them, and even where, how, and when you sleep, all play a role in the choices you make. In turn, your environment affects your stress levels, your concentration, your efficiency, and your moods. You then develop belief systems based on your experiences with your different environments. You become committed to these beliefs, which directly affects the choices you make and the results you achieve.

Is your environment negatively affecting you? Ask yourself: Do you have food allergies, skin irritations, or buzzing in the ears? Do you see spots when you close your eyes? Do you have spots on your skin, blotchiness, bloating, gas, and indigestion? Do you suffer from headaches, body aches, chronic fatigue, or tiredness? Are you irritable but don't know why? Do you have a hard time concentrating or remembering things? Do you always feel tired, but when you go to bed you can't sleep? Or, do you sleep all night, but when you wake up you just want to stay in bed and sleep more? Do you have trouble losing weight, but you can't understand why? Do you have mood swings, low energy, or memory troubles? Do you feel on edge? Do you feel like can't concentrate, feel angry for no real reason, crave stuff that you don't want to do, do stuff and don't know why, or feel all alone and have no idea where to turn?

These all could be a result of your environment and your beliefs. The good news is that by reevaluating your beliefs and following my Natural You method, you'll learn how to improve your happiness, live a healthier life, have a better career, and how to have happier, more fulfilling relationships, too. Throughout the rest of this book, you'll learn more about how your environment can affect the other 10 Keys, and how you can create an individualized plan to help you overcome what's been holding you back.

What you believe has led to the choices you've made and the lifestyle you are now living.

Key Takeaways

Your beliefs are playing the most important role in your ability to be healthy, happy, and successful long term.

The failure to distinguish what is most important to you and the beliefs you are attached to may be limiting you.

What you believe has led to the choices you've made and the lifestyle you are now living. By making changes to your beliefs, you will make the changes that will support you in letting go of unhealthy habits and behaviors.

The great thing about beliefs is that you can change them!

Continuously ask yourself, "How are my thoughts, feelings, and beliefs affecting my way of being? What beliefs are present for me? Why do I keep these beliefs? Are these beliefs supporting me to feel great? "

Your environment can affect your beliefs, and vice versa. Chronic symptoms and health problems may be a result of your environment.

Consistency has brought you to where you are right now. If you wish to experience something different, making simple little changes, tweaks, and adjustments consistently will ensure you will get to where you truly want to be long term.

"

The work environment
is very important
in determining how
enjoyable work is.

—KUMAR MANGALAM BIRLA

Your External Work Environment

I will say it again: your internal and external environments significantly affect all aspects of you. They affect your stress levels and how your able to deal with that stress. Your environments affect whether your body or mind are dealing with chronic ailments and issues, or whether they are powerful enough to eliminate them. These environments determine if your relationships are happy or not. They affect whether you achieve high levels of success and support you to maintain it, or whether you consistently deal with frustration and failure. And, they most definitely can enhance your satisfaction with life or create a space where your body and mind are in protection mode. Your choice of environment also directly impacts whether or not you live a life of joy, harmony, happiness, creation, peace, and fulfillment.

> Your choice of environment also directly impacts whether or not you live a life of joy, harmony, happiness, creation, peace, and fulfillment.

The environments you create for yourself or choose to spend your time in have a dramatic impact on your happiness, health, and the success of your business, your family, and your overall life. Reflecting on the environments you experience—and the internal environments you create based on beliefs and choice—will open your mind to understanding the changes you can make to live the extraordinary life that you love. Or, of course, you are free to choose to continue to live how you always have.

> **If you grew up with your parents telling you that you'd be happiest in a nice, safe middle-management J-O-B, and you bought into that belief, making it your own, and you followed that path, chances are you'll never make it to the C-Suite, start your own business, or travel the world in your own rock band, even if those careers would ultimately make you happier.**

Your beliefs drive your perception and choices, which shape your environment and your experiences. It's all intertwined. If you believe your life should be a certain way, you'll put in a lot of effort to create that life subconsciously. I see this all the time: people say they want one thing, and yet their mindset and actions show the exact opposite.

For example, if you grew up with your parents telling you that you'd be happiest in a nice, safe middle-management J-O-B, and you bought into that belief, making it your own, and you followed that path, chances are you'll never make it to the C-Suite, start your own business, or travel the world in your own rock band, even if those careers would ultimately make you happier.

And, if you do put in the effort to achieve those high-level positions or those amazing goals, the chances that you'll be able to maintain that success long term will be drastically reduced. We see this regularly in athletes, celebrities, singers, corporate CEOs . . . just about anywhere you look. Someone achieves extraordinary success, only to quickly crash and burn, often times out in public for all the world to see, many times privately and even all alone.

What you believe, you achieve! If you really want to know what your deep, subconscious beliefs are, take a good honest look at you, your body, your health, your relationships, your career, and your achievements. That is the true story of what you really believe. What you believe drives your choices, which create your environment, the life you live, the body you're living it in, and the people you share it with.

Is Your Environment Working for You?

The first step to understand how your environment is affecting your life and how it may be holding you back from being your happiest, healthiest self is to do a little exploration. You need to take a good, hard, honest look at what's surrounding you, and be honest with yourself about how it's impacting how you feel on an ongoing basis.

Start out by taking a basic survey of what's around you in your environment. Whom you are spending most of your time with, and where you are spending it all contribute to your ultimate happiness, success, and wellbeing. The choices you make, the foods you eat, the way you use your body, the rest you give yourself mentally and physically, and what you focus on can be used as a mirror to the real you that is driving your life. These all contribute to your overall environment. Take a note of how you spend each day, and how any changes to that routine affect how you feel.

Next time you walk into your work or home environment, notice how you feel when you arrive and then notice how you feel after you have been there a few hours. How does it feel, smell, and look? If you have never done this, I suggest you try it. Ask yourself:

Is your work/home environment a safe-haven for you?

- How do you feel when you are on your way to your home or office? Are you happy and excited to get there, or do you the long way around, hoping for every red light?

- How do you feel when you are at work or at home?

- Is your work/home environment a safe-haven for you? Can you completely turn off, unwind, let go, and just Be You?!

- Is it quiet, clean, organized, and comfortable?

- Is it a place you can really be the best version of yourself and feel great in?

- Does being there energize you or drain you?

- Are you inspired and supported to be the best version of you?

If you really want to be healthy, happy, and successful, it is vital to be in a place you feel great about, a place where you can truly be the *real* you, in order to be really great at being you!

Look around you and notice how you feel when in your different environments. Becoming aware of how different things affect you is a powerful step towards creating the real you. Everyone and everything affects you. Notice how you feel when you walk in a room and you remember, feel, or see someone there you don't like. How does it change your energy, your mood, and your enjoyment levels? Do you allow that to empower you or take away from your happiness? Muhammad Ali stated, "I win or lose a fight before I step in the ring."

Let's consider another example. After you eat a big piece of chocolate cake, how are your energy levels directly after eating the cake? What about a few hours later? How does your body feel later in the day, or the next day? How is your mind performing?

> If you really want to be healthy, happy, and successful, it is vital to be in a place you feel great about, a place where you can truly be the *real* you, in order to be really great at being you!

When you choose to share your time and invest your energy, be aware of your attitude and demeanor in each situation, whether it be doing something on your own or with others, spending time with someone eating, drinking, taking something, going somewhere, or talking or thinking about something. How are you affected before going and while you are there? How is your energy effected while you are there? Notice how you feel after a few hours, and maybe even the next day.

When you make the time to appreciate how everything affects everything, it will become a big indicator of whether the choices you are making are giving to or taking away from what you really want in your life and business.

When I guide people through the 10 Keys to Ultimate Health, Happiness, and Success, environment becomes fundamental to achieve the results they are looking for. When exploring this area of your life, it's also important to distinguish between *external environments*, like where you work and live and the people you spend time with, and *internal environments*, which are impacted by your perception, the way you see things, what you focus on, and your beliefs. These things all directly affect the choices you make, including the foods you eat and the products and the pharmaceuticals you use. Your external and internal environments can either enhance or deplete you; it's your choice. In the next few sections we'll explore this difference, looking at some practical ways to create healthy environments that are in tune with who you are and that help you achieve your goals.

> When you make the time to appreciate how everything affects everything, it will become a big indicator of whether the choices you are making are giving to or taking away from what you really want in your life and business.

Your External Work Environment

Our office environments, and the individuals we work with and for, impact our natural selves. Most of the time we are unaware of this fact. But, you should be acutely aware of the effects your environment is having on your productivity and career, which ultimately affect your health and your life. Your work environment could be holding you back from your greatest potential, performance, and success. Whether you commute to an office or work from home, you need a healthy environment to achieve the extraordinary results I am proposing in this book.

It's easy to get stressed when you have a boss or investors keeping you under the gun, co-workers or staff who are difficult to communicate with, or work in a cubicle with no windows (and let's not forget how stressful working from home can be). But, most of us tend to underestimate the extensive effects that all of that stress can cause. When you work in sub-optimal surroundings, the work you produce will be sub-optimal as well.

So how do you overcome a bad work environment, or how do you start to change it? The first step you should take is to take a good, hard, honest look at what surrounds you, both physically and emotionally. When evaluating your work environment, here are some things to consider:

- Do you have an enjoyable and peaceful journey to work? Or, do you find yourself already frustrated when you arrive? What role did your perception have?

- How does being at work make you feel? What makes you feel that way?

- Do certain people you work with make you feel happy, confident, and supported?

- Does anyone make you feel stressed, anxious, and unable to perform at the levels you know you could or would like to?

- What changes would make your work environment healthier and more efficient so you can feel empowered and supported in your success?

- Do you love what you do? Are you passionate about doing it every day?

Knowing the answers to these questions will help you begin to understand how you can change your environment so you can work more efficiently, and possibly even finally make that tough step to totally remove yourself from a toxic environment that you don't want to be in anyway.

The Natural You approach considers environment *the second most important contributor* to becoming and maintaining the best version of you long term. Since many spend the majority of the day and week in an office, we'll look at how to set up an optimal environment in the office setting.

So how do you overcome a bad work environment, or how do you start to change it?

This also applies to you if you don't have a traditional work environment, like if you're a stay-at-home parent, self-employed, or don't work in an office at all. You are affected by your surroundings at home, possibly even more so than someone who works outside of the home. If you have children, you also have the very important role of being a parent who educates that little soul to learn how to make wise life and health choices so they can grow into being a healthy, happy and successful individual, one who will also teach their kids how to be healthy, happy and successful.

When becoming aware of your environment, use all five senses. I start with my eyes closed. I feel, listen, and smell. When I open my eyes, I focus on the initial impact I sense. Did I feel instantly happy, stressed, ashamed, excited, scared, shocked, sad, frustrated, or depressed? How is the lighting? Is the area bright, relaxing, natural, and empowering, or is it dark and gloomy? The lighting in your home, the products you use to clean your home, where your home is located, your furniture (especially your bed), your air quality, water quality, the colors you use, pictures you have, the way your environment is decorated, and whether you even like your home to begin with all affect every aspect of you.

Creating Your Environmental Office

An 'environmental office' is an office that is, wherever it may be, conducive to you performing your daily tasks in a highly energized way. It is an office that helps you achieve your short- and long-term goals, and one that is healthy for you, too. To be the best you can be and maintain it long term, you must be in environments that empower you, enhance your natural talents, encourage you to do better, and create a sense of fulfillment and achievement.

> In fact, when you learn how to use stress to your advantage, stress becomes a very powerful support in pushing you outside of your comfort zone.

Negative stress has a profound effect on your health. The worst part is, often we don't realize we are negatively stressed until we get sick "all of a sudden." Negative stress has a huge effect on your entire body and mind, including your immune system. When you're negatively stressed, your body produces a hormone called cortisol. Cortisol suppresses your immune system, which means you get sick more often, and more severely. It also directly impacts your efficiency, concentration, and performance levels. So, if you've downplayed the effects of negative stress before, I hope you won't in the future. Making a few small adjustments now to create an empowering environmental office will noticeably help you become better at being you now, and can keep you healthy in the future.

Your environmental office needs to be one that works in balance with your mental environment, your home environment, and your beliefs. Remember, your beliefs affect your choices, which directs your lifestyle, which affects your health, which affects your performance which has a dramatic effect on everything, including how much money you earn, how others view you, your relationships, happiness, and so on. Yes, stress is necessary and a natural part of our life. In fact, when you learn how to use stress to your advantage, stress become a very powerful support in pushing you outside of your comfort zone. That, in turn, can catapult you to achieve beyond your goals, and help you create a bunch of exciting new ones.

However, not putting yourself first, not empowering yourself, and allowing stress to negatively affect you will lead to endless negative issues, such as weight gain, tiredness, excessive cravings, concentration trouble, mood swings, overthinking, bad choices, unexpected diagnoses and diseases. Overbearing negative stress should be considered a pandemic these days. It's shocking how many people are walking around suffering and have no idea their suffering could be caused by their perception, beliefs, environment, lifestyle, relationships, and/or career choices.

The physical space you work in is also a very important part of your environmental office. Is your 'office space' set up to support you, assist you, encourage you, and empower you? Do you have what you need where you need it? Do you have the support you need, physically and emotionally, to be doing your job better than anyone else? It doesn't matter what your J-O-B is. Whether you're a toilet bowl cleaner or the king of a country, if you stand out as awesome, that will encourage self-growth, fulfillment, and endless possibilities.

If you have no passion or excitement for the way you spend your time, if you don't bother to put your best into whatever it is you are doing, if you stop or change your life for others and consistently ignore and stifle the real you, then how can you expect to feel great and live an exceptional life?

> It's shocking how many people are walking around suffering and have no idea their suffering could be caused by their perception, beliefs, environment, lifestyle, relationships, and/or career choices.

If someone else is observing you and you're not performing your duties well, when the opportunity arises for more work, a promotion, a partnership opportunity, the right relationship opportunity, or any other life-changing opportunity, do you think you will be offered that opportunity, or if you are offered the opportunity, how well do you think that will work out long term, if you are not in the right mental and physical condition to maintain it long term?

When others think of your work or personal ethic, do they hold you in high regard, and get excited about the opportunity to explore more options with you? Or, do they wonder about you and have concerns that you don't really care, or that you're not the type of person they want to share their time, money or energy with?

> If you have no passion or excitement for the way you spend your time, if you don't bother to put your best into whatever it is you are doing, if you stop or change your life for others and consistently ignore and stifle the real you, then how can you expect to feel great and live an exceptional life?

Ask yourself: if you could see you from others' perspective, would you hire you, give you a promotion, go on a date with you, or ask you to join in a life-changing opportunity?

Here is a great saying by Sir Winston Churchill: *"To each there comes in their lifetime a special moment when they are figuratively tapped on the shoulder and offered the chance to do a very special thing, unique to them and fitted to their talents. What a tragedy if that moment finds them unprepared or unqualified for that which could have been their finest hour."*

Tips to Create Your Best Environmental Office

BE ORGANIZED.

Being disorganized is one habit that will cause more negative stress and make you less productive. Not only is being in a messy environment generally stressful, but your inability to find anything or work efficiently because of your disorganization will make you even more stressed out, whether you believe it or not. You'll end up in a vicious cycle, spiraling downward to poor health mentally, emotionally, and eventually physically.

> When you've planned well, you'll be more relaxed, you'll enjoy traveling more, and you'll be more productive on your trip.

If you travel for work, you need to be even more organized. Make sure you have what you need, where you need it, when you need it. Pre-planning and organizing ensures efficiency and productivity, which support a clear and powerful mind. Knowing what you're going to be doing as you travel and what you need to have in place or with you while you travel and spend time away is the best way to ensure you maintain a great mental and physical state throughout the journey. When you've planned well, you'll be more relaxed, you'll enjoy traveling more, and you'll be more productive on your trip.

> When you learn to include fun into pretty much everything you do, your life becomes so much better for you and everyone involved with you, and everything you're doing benefits.

HAVE FUN.

You must include fun in your environment. Put funny quotes or pictures of great memories in your folder and desk drawers. Put them on your computer, or wherever else you look frequently. There is not much available that is more powerful then opening a folder during a stressful meeting or difficult time and seeing a goofy picture that makes you laugh every time you see it. It instantly takes you from a mental place of stress or negativity to a calm and happy mind. That picture will bring you to a mind that is able to think more clearly and focus better.

When you learn to include fun into pretty much everything you do, your life becomes so much better for you and everyone involved with you, and everything you're doing benefits.

SET YOURSELF UP FOR SUCCESS

Use this checklist to maintain a healthy environmental office:

- Make sure you have what you need, where you need it, and when you need it in order to do whatever you are going to do, so that you can do it better than anyone else.

- Put great energy, passion, and fun into everything you do. When you live life this way, everything will change!

- If you work in an office, put your most important (most often turned to) documents, folders, tools, and so on within easy reach. Can you walk into your office, in the dark, and find what you need?

- Keep tools, supplies, and anything else you need where you can easily access them when you need them, and remember to put them back immediately after you use them.

- Put items around your work area that make you smile and inspire you. This includes framed photographs of loved ones, "Bucky Toys," pictures of your goals and dreams, and so on.

- Declutter your space (donate, keep, discard); use this method to eliminate any unnecessary items in your workspace.

- Use an ergonomic keyboard for your computer and an ergonomic chair to sit in for long hours. (My clients sit on a big exercise ball rather than a chair. Don't laugh—try it for a week and see how you feel).

- Use tinted screen covers for computer screens, or specially-tinted glasses (if you wear glasses), to help prevent eyesight irritation.

- Apply essential oils around you or purchase a small diffuser. Aromatherapy does wonders for stress management.

- Make sure the colors in your space make you feel good, and avoid dark, drab colors.

- Add living plants to your space—it will add life to your environmental office.

- Create a vision board on your wall (or in your folder, case, or screensaver) with pictures of things that you enjoy, goals you have, and places you want to go.

- Put your long-term and short-term goals where you can see them, as well as acknowledgments of goals you have already achieved.

- Set a nice-sounding timer on your phone every few hours to remind you to get up and move. Movement improves concentration, lowers stress, and nourishes the body's need to move. It will also help to alleviate niggling aches and pains. If you have a stairway nearby, use it. Take a couple of minutes every 1.5–2 hours and walk or run up and down the stairs.

- Get into the natural light regularly, and into the sunshine if you can. Yes, the sun is good for you—enjoy it. Even doing this for 60 seconds every hour will make a remarkable improvement in your day. Try it and see for yourself.

- If you have a hard decision to make or you're dealing with a nasty person, excuse yourself for 60 seconds. Do a walk around the office or go up and down the stairs. Get your face in the sunshine, close your eyes, take a deep breath and enjoy it, even for a few seconds. Then, go back to what you were doing and see how clear your mind feels and how much better you handle the situation.

- Set a reminder to ensure you eat at least every two hours. When I say eat, I don't mean a chocolate bar, energy bar, sandwich, coffee, energy drink, or anything else pre-packaged or processed. Eat something fresh. If you have an issue with energy, weight, concentration, memory, or mood swings, try eating fresh, unprocessed food every hour and a half to two hours for a day and see how different you feel.

- Drink water. Keep a glass bottle of water by you all day. (Make sure it is not in the direct sun.) Get into the habit of sipping on it all day. Take small sips, a mouthful at a time. If you're running to the bathroom all day, you are either drinking too fast or you're dehydrated. If you are not used to drinking water all day, it will take a while for your body to adapt. Be patient and give it a few days. When you sip water all day, you will enjoy countless benefits, including more energy, weight loss, better concentration, better memory, and fewer food cravings. See Chapter 9 for my recommendations on what you should add to your water daily.

Make your office space a place where you feel good and you will perform at your best. Your 'creation' space should be a harmonious space that inspires and empowers you. This checklist is one tool you can use to turn a career that feels draining into something exceptional. It will also give you the time and space to consider following a career path you absolutely love. Getting paid to do something you love will be a source of freedom, happiness, and success—I know from personal experience.

> ## What could you achieve if you were really present in your life, if you were not running on automatic, but were clearly choosing to do what encouraged, supported, and empowered you to do what you do to the best of your ability?

DON'T BE AFRAID TO MAKE BIG CHANGES

What should you do if changing your environment doesn't help? If you follow the guidelines here to improve your workspace and you still hate your work where you're doing your work, or the way you are doing your work, then it may be time to make a move to a new job or a new career.

Why continue doing something you don't enjoy in a place you don't like being? Your life is your choice. You can choose to make it as good or as bad as you want. As one of my mentors and favorite actors, Bill Murray, says, "This is not a dress rehearsal, this is your life." What could you achieve if you were really present in your life, if you were not running on automatic, but were clearly choosing to do what encouraged, supported, and empowered you to do what you do to the best of your ability?

Key Takeaways:

Your environment has a massive impact on your health and happiness. If your work or home environment are not supporting and encouraging you, they're holding you down and back.

Your environment can lead to everything from more frequent colds to weight gain to chronic health problems to failed relationships and dreams.

What you believe drives your choices, which create your environment, the life you live, the body you're living it in, and the people you're sharing your life with.

You *must* take the time to evaluate your internal and external environment to understand how they are affecting you. Sometimes these evaluations are difficult and uncomfortable, but they are crucial if you really want to live the life you dream of.

Your work environment can make you wildly successful or totally miserable. If your career isn't going like you want it to, take a good hard look at the environment in which you work, your beliefs, choices, and actions. When you choose to be the best version of you and to do everything to the best of your ability, endless opportunities will come your way.

"

Everything around you,
especially your home
environment, mirrors
your inner self. So
by changing your home,
you also change
the possibilities in
your own life.

—KAREN KINGSTON

Creating a "Heart-Healthy" Home Environment

Your body is sensitive to every little nuance of your circumstantial environment, whether you are aware of it or not. If "home is where the heart is," then you want a heart-healthy home. Your home is *the* most important place in your life and has the *biggest* impact on your health, happiness, and overall success. This includes the lifestyle choices of all the people living with you, the air and water quality in your home, the products and furnishings you bring into your home, your energy usage, and everything down to your bedding choices.

Unfortunately, most people don't understand and believe how much of an impact their home has on their health. Even tidy, domestically-oriented people often don't consider the things that matter most with regards to creating a healthy home environment. Recall that your body is sensitive to every little nuance of your circumstantial environment.

> If "home is where the heart is," then you want a heart-healthy home.

If you don't like what surrounds you at home, if anything and everything from the people to the décor to the layout of your home doesn't support great health, high levels of natural energy, and feelings of safety, relaxation, and happiness, then your home adds to negativity in your life, and it takes away from your positive intentions. That additional tension weighs on you, taking its toll both emotionally and physically. Even though things like your furniture or paint or art choices seem minimal, they really can have a bigger impact on your life and your health.

How do you begin to create a home environment that's good for your health? Simply be more aware of the choices you can make to create an environmentally-friendly home. It will not only make an enormous impact on the quality of life and health you and your family have, but it can also completely enhance and improve all your relationships. I am not talking about installing solar panels or a wind turbine on your property (although they might be good ideas, too). It's simply about creating a healthy, happy, empowering home environment that you look forward to being in and love to be in.

Who Created Your Home Environment?

Committing yourself to creating an empowering, tranquil, and harmonious home is a very empowering and liberating experience. It can be done by yourself if you live alone, or, if you live with others, with your partner's and/or children's help. Remember, a healthy, loving home is created by *all* the people who live in it. I am often surprised when a client tells me that they have a healthy, loving home but their partner is always miserable and they argue all the time in the house. When I visit their home, it all makes perfect sense. The environment is clearly created with little or no input from the other person or people living there.

> A home that excludes or belittles the wants, needs, personality, and energy of those living there is unlikely to encourage anyone living there to be happy or healthy.

A home should be set up and laid out for *everyone* living there, with everyone's input and everyone's personalities shining. If you do not feel great in your home, ask yourself why. If your family doesn't love being together in the home, ask them why, and really listen. If you have decorated, designed, organized, and created your "family home" all on your own—making all the where, what, and how choices—or if someone else did it for you, it is not surprising that you or your partner don't love being there. If you believe you have "awesome" taste and your partner's taste is "terrible" and you decide that you're going to do it your way, you have essentially created an "alone home" that's not centered around the entire family. That means anyone who lives in the home but does not feel a part of the home will not feel supported, encouraged, loved, wanted, or needed there. Why would they be happy and healthy there?

When I am invited to analyze a client's home, I often ask the same question: "Where is your partner's input in this home?" Nine times out of ten I get a little smirk or giggle, a roll of the eyes, a deep breath and negative comment about their partner's "taste." Is this a harmonious, loving, family home? No, it is not. If you want to share your life with someone else and you want your partner to feel loved and respected, then you must include that person in all aspects of your life and together home, or eventually you will be alone again.

Whoever may have won the battle about how your home looks and feels may feel good about what they created, but essentially, they have lost in the bigger picture of the happy, healthy, and loving home in a mutually-respected relationship. A home that excludes or belittles the wants, needs, personality, and energy of those living there is unlikely to encourage anyone living there to be happy or healthy. For children to be happy, healthy, and successful, it is also essential for them to live in a congruent, relaxed, healthy home with happy parents who are in love, and who love spending time together. To support your relationship, it is vital that you make the space and regularly schedule the time for you and your partner, not just as parents, but as partners and lovers. When you as a couple have a powerful, loving bond, your family will have the strong foundation it needs to grow and thrive in all ways. Your children will feel secure, and everyone in the family will be on the right road to an exceptional life.

Making your together home an important focus of your daily life will improve the lives of everyone in the family. When everyone enjoys what they're surrounded by, they'll feel more happy and relaxed, which improves the dynamic of the entire family. And, it will have a powerful impact on everyone's happiness, health, and success now and long into the future.

Assessing Your Own Home

Remember, all five senses are affected by your surroundings. Take a step back and start by entering your home. When you first walk up to your front door, and when you open your door to walk in, close your eyes and analyze. Listen and smell, feel the energy in your home. Ask a real friend for their advice on what your home looks, sounds, feels, and smells like. (Make sure you ask a real, healthy, happy, successful friend, one who isn't envious or negative, and is someone you admire.) Look around—does it make you feel good and bring a sense of calm and happiness? Are you grateful to be there? Do you think, "Ahhhh, I'm home," with a smile on your face, or do you feel tense, anxious, disappointed, and frustrated?

> **When you can just stop, turn off completely, and just be you with no pressure or stress, then you are home.**

When my friends come to my homes to lay around and relax, they almost always fall asleep straight away. I love it! I always believed if people sat on my couch and passed out, without having consumed too much of anything, but because my home was so calm and relaxing, it must be a great place to be. When you can just stop, turn off completely, and just be you with no pressure or stress, then you are home.

You can also try the following test:

1. How do you feel when you are driving home?
   a. You are excited to get home and want to get there ASAP.
   b. You take a long way home, maybe making a pit stop or two.

2. How do you feel when you arrive home?
   a. You are excited to get in the house, rushing to meet those who are waiting for you, and they are excited that you are there.
   b. You sit in the car, take deep breaths, listen to the radio, or play on your phone, taking some quiet time to prepare yourself.

3. **When you first open your front door and walk into your home, take 10 seconds to close your eyes and take a deep breath.** How does your home welcome you?
   a. "I love being home."
   b. "I don't feel great here."

4. **How does your home look (to you, considering your needs and wants)?**
   a. Relaxing and welcoming
   b. Tense—it stresses you out

If you chose (a) for every answer, fantastic. If you chose (b), why? And how long will you wait to change it?

Why would you choose to be where you don't feel great? And if you are living in a home that makes you feel less than great, how is that affecting every other aspect of your life? Is the added stress of spending so much time in a home that you dislike affecting your health? Are you getting sick more often than you should? Or, are you just generally grumpy, in a bad mood, or even depressed? Ask yourself, "What can I do to make my home feel so good that I look forward to spending time here, and so that when I am here I am able to repair, recharge, and inspire my soul?"

Now, ask your partner and/or children the same questions, and really, truly, openly, and lovingly *listen* to the answers, without interrupting, and with the desire to understand clearly. See if they give the same answers that you feel. Remember that their opinions and input as unique and valued individuals are vital to the dynamics of your entire family. They deserve to live in a home that makes them feel safe, comfortable, encouraged, empowered, and happy. If you learn that they don't enjoy being in your home, then you need to question why you have not changed these aspects of your home, or whether or not you even want them there.

Your surroundings severely affect your relationship with your family and the way everyone feels about that relationship. If going home, arriving home, setting foot in your home, and being at home doesn't make you happy, how can you possibly have happy, healthy relationships there? Conversely, if being at home makes you feel relaxed and at peace, empowered, respected, and supported, imagine how that feeling will translate to how you interact with your family members and partner, and how they interact with you. Your home could be a sanctuary for everyone living there, if you would just choose to make it that way.

The Importance of High-Quality Drinking Water

Your healthy home goes beyond how you decorate it or how it smells. It even goes beyond the feeling you get when you walk over the threshold into your home. There are tests you can do in your home environment to make it more "heart-healthy." Two important factors to analyze are air and water quality.

> One of the top, most important, most valuable things you can invest in to empower a healthy body is to ensure you have pure, clean, natural, energized water.

Did you know drinking poor-quality water—i.e., water infused with fluoride and chlorine—is responsible for an increase in bladder and rectal cancer, breast cancer, asthma, gastrointestinal disease, obesity, mood swings and a host of other immune issues? Moreover, lead in water can result in severe developmental delays and/or learning disorders in children, as well as anxiety and memory and concentration issues. Long term, it can cause issues such as Alzheimer's and dementia. This is true not only for drinking water, but all the water in your home, whether it's for washing your laundry, showering and bathing, or cleaning and cooking. Your body is made of up to 78% water, depending on your age and lifestyle choices. The cleaner that water is, the better all areas of your life will be.

When it comes to water quality in your home, one of the top, most important, most valuable things you can invest in to empower a healthy body is to ensure you have pure, clean, natural, energized water. We live on a planet that is full of toxins and all sorts of other stuff that be detrimental to your health. The government is adding all kinds of stuff into our water sources, and big business is dumping all sorts of pollutants into our water, too. Plus, the old water pipes and lines your water has to run through long before it even gets to your tap can leach toxins into your drinking water, too. Drinking water from your tap or pre-bottled from some big business is creating one of the biggest health issues on the planet.

> If there is one most important thing you need for the rest of your life, it's pure clean water in your home.

There are many really interesting tests being carried out about the importance of water and your relationship with it. I strongly urge you to do a little research on this for yourself because it has big implications. Remember that awareness and assessing your beliefs is one of the 10 Keys to Ultimate Happiness, Success, and Health. You may also enjoy the amazing work by Dr. Masaru Emoto on the Hado effect.[1][2] Dr. Emoto's work showed that the energy that is put into water affects how the water molecules behave. His books will open your eyes to the importance of water in your life.

It is an absolute must to have pure water in your house. If you are broke, even if you can't afford new shoes, then I say start saving. Skip your daily coffee, forget about the chocolate treats, fast food lunches, cigarettes, and start scraping together money for a good water filter. If there is one most important thing you need for the rest of your life, it's pure clean water in your home. Put it right at the top of your 'must have' list and get it as soon as possible. Start drinking pure, clean water and you will notice big changes overnight.

You can install water filters on all the faucets and shower heads if you live in a municipal area. If you live rurally and collect water from a well, you may want to have the water tested to see if it is "heavy" or "hard" water, and to see what types of bacteria, toxins, and other harmful substances may have worked their way into your well water. If there is anything in the water that should be removed, do what you can to improve the quality and healthfulness of the supply right before use.

Even just using a filtration pitcher for drinking and cooking water can help. As long as you buy a high-quality filter and change its filter cartridges often, you'll see results. Or, even better, save up and install

---

[1] Emoto, M. (2011). *The hidden messages in water.* Simon and Schuster.

[2] Emoto, M. (2011). *The secret life of water.* Simon and Schuster.

Reg's Natural Home Tweaks

1. Invest in you. The money you use to get a high-quality reverse osmosis and water ionizer for all your drinking, cooking, and washing water will pay for itself in the reduced costs of maintenance and cleaning supplies, plus all the health benefits. Your body and mind will love you for it over the long term, too.

2. Get a central reverse osmosis unit installed to clean all the water throughout the rest of the home. It will save you money on everything from pipes and fittings to cleaning supplies. You will be amazed at the power of pure, clean water! It will keep you and your home clean naturally. Did you know you can even degrease your oven with pure water? Pure clean water will eliminate the need for harmful and expensive chemical cleaners.

3. Air quality is affected by many factors, including off-gassing from products and furnishings, through to the materials and equipment, to the windows, doors, and ventilation system you have in your house. You should have regular maintenance done on your vents and replace your air filters regularly to keep them clean. I always recommend having an HVAC specialist come to your home and give you an honest assessment of your current HVAC systems and units. You will be surprised at what you learn. Become aware of smells like chemicals, molds, plastic, cleaners, and such, and do all you can to eliminate and neutralize them naturally.

4. Invest in a great vacuum cleaner, one that has very strong suction, even if the bag is full. Make sure your vacuum cleaner is sucking up and trapping, all the dirt and dust it sucks in, not just sucking it in one end and blowing it out the other. And, put a few drops of your favorite pure, organic essential oil in the filter to detox your air.

5. Invite lots of live, big green leafy plants into your home and have fun regularly using aromatherapy with the purest essential oils you can find. Grow your own herbs and veggies, too. It's a great way to learn about your food, explore new flavors, relax your mind, enhance your home's energy, and re-oxygenate your air all at the same time.

a whole-house, complete reverse osmosis system right where the water comes in your home and a water ionizer for your drinking and cooking water. I suggest a top-quality complete reverse osmosis unit combined with an ionizer, either for your entire home or, at a minimum, for the water you use to drink and cook with.

How Clean is the Air in Your Home?

What about the air you are breathing when in your home? Numerous studies have now shown that indoor air pollution is a greater threat to your health than outdoor air pollution. This includes stale and stagnant air, toxic fumes, off-gassing, tobacco smoke, cleaning supplies, dust mites, mold and mildew, pollen, household sprays, and even perfumes. Remember, we learned a while back in the book about energy and how everything affects everything. Imagine now adding all that energy to all the household toxins, and how that combination could possibly be affecting you.

The things that you use to fill your house can be even more dangerous. Your furniture (including your mattress!), your kids' toys, and anything else that has that 'new' smell could be off gas dangerous chemicals that can harm your health. When you get new furniture, home décor items, toys, or anything else you place in your home, chances are they've been made with fire-retardant and other chemicals. Anything made from plastic will also off gas dangerous compounds. Those chemicals leech out into the air (and onto your skin) where they can make impact your performance, or worse, make you sick.

You've probably heard that underactive thyroid is a big problem for many people, and that it can cause big problems with weight gain. You may even have a friend or two who have an underactive thyroid. It's almost epidemic in the United States right now. Did you know that the chemicals that off gas from the stuff in your home can lead to underactive thyroid? Studies have linked the rise of hypothyroidism to the introduction of flame retardant chemical applications to furniture cushions and fabrics, clothing, electronics and so on. While the original intent was to prevent injury and death, it turns out that the chemicals are absorbed into our bodies where they can cause a lot of harm. There's probably a lot that you're not aware of when it comes to air quality.

It's especially important to pay attention to the things you're bringing into your home if you're pregnant, or if you plan to become pregnant. The fire-retardant chemicals that are used in the manufacture of many household items can terribly harm a developing fetus. These chemicals have been shown to increase prenatal mortality rates, as well as increasing the risk of a whole suite of birth defects. These chemicals can amplify problems with anatomical development in the nervous system, cardiovascular system, respiratory system, and just about every other major body system.[3]

> Numerous studies have now shown that indoor air pollution is a greater threat to your health than outdoor air pollution.

Hundreds of thousands of people fall ill to air-related disease every year, while others are suffering from endless other diseases from household and personal products. Rather than getting to the core of all these health issues that are caused by an overload of toxic stuff all around us, what is the usual course of action? More drugs!

When it comes to air quality in your home, clean it regularly. The easiest and nicest way to do this is naturally. Keep your windows open just a little. Invite live plants into your home. (Notice I said "invite." If your plants keep dying, ask yourself, "Do I love them? Do I want them here? Do I take time to love them and give them what they need?") Plants are living things and need to be cherished. Researchers have done endless tests on the energy and behavior of plants and found that plants react to actions and energy just like other living things. It has been shown that if you walk past a plant and hit it intentionally, the next time you walk past it, it will recoil away from you. There are some great videos on YouTube about it. How you feel about your plants probably determines how you treat them, and that might also be a sign of how you treat other people in your home, or outside of your home, too. If your plants and relationships are dying, take an honest look at how you treat them.

Another great way to improve your air quality, environment, energy, and health is to use medical-grade, pure, organic essential oils every day.

---

[3] United States Environmental Protection Agency. (2017). Integrated Risk Information System. Retrieved from https://www.epa.gov/iris

You can either put a couple drops around the home, in the vents, in the laundry, in the vacuum filter, in the bath, or use non-heating diffusers. I put essential oils in my laundry and in the filter of my vacuum, as well as on cotton balls to use in the car, on the airplane, or wherever I am. As there are seemingly endless oils and oil blends to choose from, have some fun with it and experiment with different ones. You can completely change your home environment into a place of balance, peace, fun, and romance just by using different oils.

If your plants and relationships are dying, take an honest look at how you treat them.

Home Improvements to Start Making Now

I have already provided some tips about making a home better for family relationships, health, and life. But what about the repairs, maintenance costs, and utility bills that are also part of your home life? Did you ever think taking steps to regain control over your utility bills and household repairs could lead you to have less stress and improved wellbeing? A healthy home environment is not only aesthetically pleasing and physically comfortable, but also economically efficient.

It's important to take care of your home for the same reasons it is vital to take care of your body. If your home is sick, or not feeling very good, it cannot be the best version of a home, meaning, it cannot serve you and provide everything you need to be healthy and happy. If you are stressed out over high energy bills or household repair expenses, and you know there is a ton of stuff that needs to be done, that worry is always taking up a bit of space in your mind so that you remember to do it one day. You cannot maintain optimal health mentally and emotionally if you're constantly worried about your home or bills. (Remember how poor health in those areas affects your body's systems and your personality.) Small home improvements can have a big impact on the cost of living in your home and your enjoyment of being there, as well as how much it costs to keep you healthy. That, in turn, can have a big impact on your happiness, stress levels, and your bank account balance.

Here are suggestions to improve different areas of your home, with respect to your health:

- **Windows and doors.** Customized windows and doors with double-pane or even triple-pane glazed glass components can do wonders. Not only can you make your home interior much more comfortable and energy efficient, but you can also keep out bugs, allergens, mold, and so on. Your energy and repair or maintenance bills will go down as these structures lock in heat in the winter and cool air in summer.

- **HVAC.** You may be able to update your units and your systems so that they are as energy efficient as possible. For example, switch to using clean air air-conditioning units. I suggest looking into the units that give you the option of incorporating essential oils into the system, so you detox and empower your air too. There are endless varieties and blends to turn your house into a home.

  Don't shy away from paying the fee to have a professional to come to your home and give you an honest assessment of your current HVAC systems and units. Remember how much the air quality in your home can affect your health and success. The little you spend now will pay for itself many times over. Your HVAC is a critical part of your home's air quality.

- **Bedding.** Your bed is at the top of my list since your body is in full-on repair and recharge mode when you are sleeping. Uncomfortable beds and pillows rob you of much-needed restful sleep, and they can cause all sorts of problems. Your mattresses should be soft but flat and supportive without lumps, bumps, or springs sticking up into your back. If possible, buy a bed and pillows made from all-natural products or at least a contour bed with at least 6" natural memory foam top with matching contour pillows. Remember how dangerous off gassing is. When you buy new, ensure you have a lot of fresh air flow through your room, lots of big green leafy plants, and that you consistently use pure essential oils in a cool diffuser near you to ensure you are neutralizing all those toxins and chemicals.

  If the air you are breathing is full of toxic fumes off gassing from chemical cleaners used to wash your sheets and pillow cases, and your bed and pillows are made from toxic materials which off gas even more chemicals, your body and mind are being poisoned while you sleep. These chemicals cause all sorts of issues: underactive thyroid, skin irritations, eczema, allergies, asthma, concentration and memory problems, mood swings, snoring, restless sleep, insomnia, and so much more. Remember to keep your bed mattress, bed sheets, and pillow cases clean to prevent illness and strong allergic reactions. Replace sheets and pillowcases with clean ones at least every second day. Make sure that they have been washed with just a little natural cleanser in pure water, and rinsed really well. (Avoid the brand names with heavy chemical compounds.)

• **Electronics.** The electronics in your house should be as modern and energy-efficient as you can afford. Every two years, see what electronics in your home can be upgraded, updated, or removed. Use direct wire plug systems as much as you can to cut down on the Wi-Fi and energy waves around your home. Make sure your electronic devices are plugged into certified outlets and extension leads are not damaged. Don't have computers, TVs, cell phones, or any other transmitting devices beside your bed or within 10 feet of your sleeping area.

• **Lights.** Energy-efficient light bulbs and lamps keep your electric bill and bulb replacement bills down and reduce stress. Your home's interior lighting should be bright but not glaring. Place lights in strategic, practical areas such as above your kitchen countertops and in corners above or next to furnishings for reading. Try replacing electric lights with candles, especially for the last two hours before bed. Avoid screen time right before bed as well; the blue light that our devices emit can keep you from falling asleep quickly. When you implement these changes, your environment will feel so much better, you will sleep better, and your monthly electric bill will go down. It's a win/win/win situation.

• **De-clutter.** A cluttered home doesn't make for a happy home interior. Even if you do have a cluttered home but don't notice any ill effects on your health, you will be amazed at how much better you feel after you make your home more organized by de-cluttering it. If you haven't used something at least once within the past year, get rid of it. You don't need it if you don't use it. Clearing out the old makes room for the new, and it will help keep you brain healthy and active.

Make sure you have plenty of fresh air, clean spaces, big living plants, happy pictures, and things to remind you of happy times to create the heart-healthy home of your dreams.

Choose Your Household Products Carefully

We've discussed the importance of air and water quality, your environment, and how the energy in your home are all affected by who and what you bring into your home. And, you have learned there are choices you can make that put the power back into your hands when it comes to your energy and house maintenance bills. Another important heart-healthy home tip that I hinted at earlier is to stop using harmful household products.

> While taking control of your health can be fun, taking control of everything you choose to put on your skin, in your body, carry around all day, and absorb into you will truly empower you.

Many household products that most people use on a daily basis contain toxic ingredients that can cause an array of health risks. They can disrupt our ability to reproduce, disrupt children's ability to develop properly, disrupt our hormones, contribute to weight gain, mood swings, and cause rashes and respiratory issues, amongst other issues. There are also chemicals used daily that are wreaking havoc on our wildlife and ending up in our water supply, ensuring everyone gets a share of the chemical, whether they use it or not.

Cutting out the toxic, chemical-laden cosmetics and cleaning products from your home and office will be a great start to lightening the toxic load on your body and in our environments. These days it's easy to find instructions for how to make your own natural, chemical-free cleaning and personal care products. It supports a more natural approach to living. While taking control of your health can be fun, taking control of everything you choose to put on your skin, in your body, carry around all day, and absorb into you will truly empower you. Putting your own energy into the foods and products you choose, will empower you in endless ways, not to mention all time and money you will save.

> Choosing the right personal care products is another incredibly important key to ensuring your body and mind are clear, clean and healthy.

Making your own products is great to do on your own, with a partner, or with your children, if you have them. It can be a lot of fun! Why not plan to make your very own household cleaning products, toothpaste, makeup, deodorants, candles and the like on the weekend? It's a great way to spend time together, and it will educate the children about all sorts of natural things and the importance of controlling what you use and bring into your home. Your family will enjoy all the positive benefits that go along with sharing time together while learning and having fun with real people. Who knows, having fun and working towards a common purpose could also open up new chapters in your relationships.

This, again, is a win/win/win situation. You can spend time with the kids or your partner or enjoy some peaceful and entertaining time all on your own. You can educate yourself and your kids on how to work with your hands, and in the process research fun, healthy, and natural ways to make the products you need, save money, detox, and clean your air. Your healthy and clean air will help to naturally detox your body— and it will give you a whole lot of other benefits. Please understand that it is vital to your home, your health, your relationships, your success, and your life to eliminate harsh chemicals from your environments and enjoy being the natural, healthy, happy, and powerful you.

Choose What You Put on Your Body Carefully

Choosing the right personal care products is another incredibly important key to ensuring your body and mind are clear, clean and healthy. Using the right products will naturally create ultimate health, happiness, and success. What you use in your environments and what you put in and on your body will determine how healthy your mind and body are. Remember, your skin is your body's largest organ. But, many of us put chemicals on our skin that we would never eat. Those chemicals negatively affect your health, no matter where or how you use them, and no matter what the safety information states.

Skin care, household cleaning, cosmetics, and other industries have regulations that are responsible for providing us with products that are "safe." But the reality is that there are more than 80,000 chemicals in use and many are unregulated. Even the regulated products state, "Do not eat me." If you shouldn't eat it, then you shouldn't put it on you either, as it gets absorbed through your skin. Forget that old myth about "not crossing the defensive blood-brain barrier" nonsense. If you shouldn't eat it, then you shouldn't breathe it in, and you shouldn't smear it all over you, either. Becoming aware of your environment and the products going in and on you is a vital step to taking control of your health and life.

Forget that old myth about "not crossing the defensive blood-brain barrier" nonsense.

A common practice you may have is using too much soap, cleaners, and laundry detergent when washing and cleaning your clothes, linens, and house. Many times, I have seen individuals with these chemicals on all day, being absorbed into their skin because they used too much, and didn't take the time to thoroughly rinse off. Have you ever put your clothes in water and watched the soap coming out of them? Imagine those chemicals being against your skin all day. Be mindful when you're cleaning your home. Don't just choose to make better cleaning products, but also make sure those products don't linger on your (or your family's) skin. Use less, and rinse more with pure water.

Most laundry detergents are full of very harmful chemicals. Unfortunately, when you do laundry, the rinse cycle often doesn't fully rinse the detergent out of your clothes, so there are still a lot of chemicals left in the fabrics. Most people wear the same clothes all day. Each outfit you change into still has chemicals in the fabric, and those chemicals stay against your skin for long periods of time. How many hours a day do you wear clothing? Do you ever sweat in them? When you sweat your clothes get wet, the chemicals become active, the pores of your skin open, and your body absorbs these chemicals. This stuff is toxic. It clearly states on the label, "Do not eat me," yet you have it on your skin all day long. Are you 'dealing with' or 'suffering from' any sort of skin issues and irritation, or any deeper organ issues? Check the soaps and cleaning supplies you use on your skin and on your clothes.

I am not trying to scare you into making a change—it is all about creating awareness. It's so important to me that you understand and become aware of how the simple changes you make in your life, like changing how you wash your clothes, can effect a positive change in the health of your skin, your organs, your mental functions, and your home. Remember, the first step toward wellness is to fully understand how your choices affect your health, and everything affects everything.

Here is another example showing how beliefs, the number one key to ultimate health, happiness, and success, plays a huge role in your choices: if a person simply believes a product is safe to use—like a pharmaceutical given to them by a doctor or a specialist, or a cleaning product used in the home every day—then they will become completely complacent and ignore the multitude of studies that prove how unsafe these chemicals are. Be aware of your beliefs, and where those beliefs came from.

Be aware of your beliefs, and where those beliefs came from.

Walk into any grocery store and find the aisle filled with processed foods, laundry detergent, and cleaners. You have plenty of choices to poison yourself with. Which one will it be? Or maybe after reading this, you may realize the facts, become more aware, and change your beliefs about these kinds of products. What are you willing to believe? You have the power to create powerful and empowering belief systems that will easily guide you to a life you love and feel great about—a life that brings you closer to being the best version of the natural you. Or, you can hold on to your old beliefs and keep doing what you have always done, so that you can keep getting more of what you've got. The choice is yours to make.

Did You Know?

- It only takes 26 seconds for the chemicals from the products you use in your home to enter the bloodstream through the air or your skin.

- There over 80,000 chemicals in use right now in the US alone, thousands of which are banned overseas.

- The air and water in your home can either ensure you have a very strong immune system and powerful mind, or they will ensure you are consistently suffering from and dealing with an endless list of issues.

> You have the power to create powerful and empowering belief systems that will easily guide you to a life you love and feel great about—a life that brings you closer to being the best version of the natural you.

Our children are at risk. Babies are born with over 200 chemicals coursing through their veins by the time they take their first breath. Studies have found more than 287 chemicals linked to issues like birth defects, developmental delays, toxicity and even cancer. Manufacturers of the cleaning products and laundry detergents you use every day to clean your home (unlike food, beverage, cosmetic, and other personal care products) are not required by federal law to list their ingredients.

Whether you are into the "green" movement or not, it is worth considering that *"we do not inherit the earth from our ancestors, we borrow it from our children."* Don't we want to leave it in better shape for them than we found it? Don't we want our children to suffer fewer health and mental issues than we do, rather than creating a life and world for them where they will be dealing with far more? Let's make a change by becoming aware of and teaching awareness to the up-and-coming generation. Let's stop polluting our bodies, our minds, the food we eat, the water we drink, the air we breathe, and the earth we enjoy living on.

I would guess that even if you do not care about the earth or how you leave it, you do care about *you*. These chemicals that are all around you *do* affect your energy, your empowerment, your body, your mind, your life, your future, your relationships, your income, your success, and your happiness. If you choose to ignore that fact, it will cost you dearly, and in more ways than you can imagine. The choice to be the best natural version of yourself starts with becoming aware of your beliefs, your choices, and your environment.

> Whether you are into the "green" movement or not, it is worth considering that *"we do not inherit the earth from our ancestors, we borrow it from our children."*

Start by choosing safer replacements to the toxic chemicals. Most large retailers sell these replacements at reasonable prices, but you can make your own like I do, for way less, or you can easily obtain the best available commercially-made products with some research online to find the best available. Natural cleaning agents and personal care products are much better for the immediate environment of your body, the external environment in your home, and the larger environment we all live in. Your clothes will last longer and your skin, teeth, hair, and eyes will be much healthier, and look better, too.

Along with natural cleaning products, there are foods and ingredients that you eat that can be used for cleaning the home. If it's safe enough for you to eat, that means it's safe to have in your environment, on your skin, and around your kids. Lemons, tea tree oil, pine oil and baking soda are just three that I use; they have been used effectively for decades with no harmful effects, and my home smells great too. Just do a Google search for 4 little words: "how to make natural," hit enter, and have fun.

If you do prefer to buy rather than making them yourself at a fraction of the cost, look for sustainable alternative replacement products that are certified Toxic-Free, Ecocert, USDA Organic, Cruelty-Free, Fair Trade, Rainforest Alliance Certified, and so on. Making these changes may seem initially hard to do, and you might think they're a waste of time, but I promise you, once you surround yourself with high-energy, natural products, you will change in ways you never knew existed. Making any change in your life is possible if you really want the benefits and results from it. A few small changes and it will become an easy normal part of your life in a very short time.

Reg's Natural You Tweaks

Choices. Take personal responsibility for your choices and your future. Become more aware of all the simple ways to make your home life healthy, happy, and empowering. Once you begin to take that on, you may find yourself throwing away a piece of trash you found on the sidewalk or you may stop buying chemical-based products from the store and start making your own natural, healthy, low cost and more effective products at home. Consider using pure, organic essential oils, live plants, find fun and tasty recipes, and begin creating a refreshingly clean, heart-healthy environment for you, your friends, and your family to enjoy.

Relationships in the Home

Here we are: the "elephant in the room." We have touched on the topic of relationships a little throughout this book, but it's important to dive a bit deeper into it. One critical area of home life I would like to look at that contributes to a heart-healthy home is the relationships you have with the people you live, eat, breathe, and sleep with. The relationships you choose to be in are one of the most powerful and important choices you will ever make. They can help you be the best version of you possible, or they can literally kill you.

> Making these changes may seem initially hard to do, and you might think they're a waste of time, but I promise you, once you surround yourself with high-energy, natural products, you will change in ways you never knew existed.

I went through a time when I was in a relationship that dragged me into the pits of depression and bad health. In fact, I was engaged to the wrong person, a woman I dedicated my heart and soul to.

I was living in London in 2010 until 2014. My life's passion was health and wellbeing, but my soul's passion was to be a husband and a father. I met a stunning lady at an event I was invited to, and she stole my heart. But then, little by little, I could feel my life force being drained out of me. My intuition and the advice from some of our friends kept telling me there was something very wrong with this relationship, and that I needed to get out, but my heart, my head, and my beliefs forced me to do all I could to "make it work." According to my upbringing and the encouragement of my mother, *relationships are about hard work and sticking with it through the good and the bad.* And, after already going through my first marriage and losing my beautiful daughters to a combination of aggressive control and endless factious rumors, I was again determined to "Make this work!"

> One critical area of home life I would like to look at that contributes to a heart-healthy home is the relationships you have with the people you live, eat, breathe, and sleep with.

My fiancé had two boys that I was crazy about, and I wanted more than anything to be a father for them. So, despite my uncertainties, I stayed with the belief I could make it better. I was fully dedicated and doing all I could. I supported them financially. I bought her a new car to ensure she was safe and able to get around. I helped look after the home. I was doing all I could to the best of my ability to be the "perfect" partner. I would take care of the kids while she was working and when we were together. I regularly drove them to school, football practice, friends' homes, and all the stuff a dad loves to do.

We would spend the evenings and weekends together as a family. When she had to go to work at night, I would make sure there was a nice hot bath and a nice home cooked meal ready for her when she got home. When she was sore or tired after dinner, I got her on the massage table to repair and relax her before bed. The house and yard were always clean and maintained, the kids were cared for, and I always made myself available to support her, listen to her, be romantic, buy her little gifts, give her funny cards, bring flowers, and always show her how much I loved and supported her. But, the relationship almost killed me.

When I found out that part of her 'business' was sleeping around with clients and 'friends' of hers, it broke me. "What was wrong with me?" I asked myself. How had I allowed myself to keep going along with such a destructive relationship against my own intuition, training, and common sense?

> Never let your beliefs overpower your intelligence. The great thing about beliefs is that "You can change them!"

It took me a long time to clear my head and my heart, and it has been one of the most powerful lessons of my life. It reinforced the importance of choice, listening to your intuition, being true to yourself, and understanding the power of environment. Here I was, a guy dedicated to health and wellbeing for himself and others. I was a guy dedicated to his relationship and the people he chose to share his life with. Yet I was ready for the grave, all because I was sharing everything I had to give with someone who had no care, concern, love, or respect for me or anyone else, and it almost destroyed me and my future.

I learned that sharing and giving of yourself is a powerful and amazing thing. It can bring you so much pleasure and take you to levels of happiness and success that you could never dream of. But, if given to the wrong people, it can be so very destructive and drag you into depths of darkness that you wouldn't wish on your worst enemy.

As you think about how to create a heart-healthy home, don't forget the most important element: the people you share it with. Listen to your gut and what it tells you, and don't let any false beliefs hold you in a relationship that negatively affects your energy, your passion, yourself, your beliefs, and your happiness, which all ultimately harm your health, or worse, could kill you.

Key Takeaways:

Make your home a 'heart-healthy' home. Your home should be a place that everyone in your family loves to spend time in, and one that reflects, supports, and empowers everyone who lives in it.

Be aware of the air and water quality inside your home. Do all you can to invest in updates and upgrades to your home so you'll always have access to the cleanest water and air.

Carefully choose the household products you use. The chemicals that you're exposed to, on a daily basis, have a huge impact on your health, especially chemicals that stay in contact with your skin.

The people you share your home with have an immense impact on your health and happiness. Make sure you choose them wisely, and listen to your intuition when it comes to your relationships.

Never let your beliefs overpower your intelligence. The great thing about beliefs is that "You can change them!"

"

Your immune cells
are like a circulating
nervous system. Your
nervous system in fact
is a circulating nervous
system. It thinks. It's
conscious

—DEEPAK CHOPRA

The Protector of Your Internal Environment— Your Immune System

I hope by now that you understand how your external world contributes to your overall wellbeing. In the next two chapters, I want to explore your internal environments. These are the environments found within your body—the cellular experience of your external world. The body is an organism made up of systems that are either working exceptionally well, functioning 'normally,' performing below average, or not working. Using my Natural You tweaks and the natural wisdom presented here in this book, you will empower and optimize your body's systems. I will dive deeper into ways you can support all your interconnected systems to function and operate in a way that leaves you feeling like the best version of you. You will discover the power of your immune system, how something as common as sugar can create dysfunction in your systems, and how you can use vitamins naturally produced in the body to create health in your life.

The Lymphatic System

Without our immune system, we would all be forced to live in sterile environments, never touching each other, feeling a spring breeze, or tasting the rain. The immune system is a complex operation within our

Testmonial

To Reg Lenney,
The one and only person who managed to change my life in just a few months.

Meeting Reg has been life changing for me. I have been suffering from an autoimmune disease and a lot of eczema since the age of 17. With a constant running in and out of hospitals and treated by specialists with adrenocortical treatments internally and externally for 30 years and in chemotherapy treatment for more or less 15 years. Most of the doctors have told me the same answer, "Just learn to live with your disease." Luckily I'm a very strong person in mind; otherwise I wouldn't have made it to the place I am now.

The constant hormone treatment provokes weight gain and bloating, which are very difficult to eliminate with a normal diet. I experienced all the possible side effects of chemotherapy known. And with an autoimmune disease follows an autoimmune depression, which has been there for all the years.

Reg has managed during the past 3.5 months to almost completely cleanse and detox my body, cells, organs even my mind has been almost cleared from all the negativity (I say almost because we haven't finished the programme yet), but I strongly believe that we will be successful....

Taking all this into consideration I'm still on chemotherapy treatment (on lowest and last dose), got separated end of December 2014, but still felt great during the whole period, and very important to me I had lost 16 kg in 7 weeks.

The normal IgE is <128 but due to my immune system disease, mine has always been extremely high at around 2000 in bad periods and between 1500-1200 in good periods of sleeping disease.

However after working with Reg for 7 weeks my IgE had decreased to 670, the doctors were amazed. At first they didn't recognize me, not only did I look healthier, my skin was much better and had lost weight, but most important of all they had never seen such a quick decrease in my blood levels for such a short period of time. I explained about my programme with Reg and they were very happy on my behalf.

On my next visit to the doctors I was down on an IgE of 520. I can now really feel the difference in my body, my behaviour, my sleep, the functioning of all the organs and my overall feeling towards *myself. As a matter of fact I was recently offered a job at the lingerie store "Agent Provocateur." Which boosted my self-confidence to an extreme that it hadn't reached in years. I loved it. On several occasions I have met friends who didn't recognize me. That also confirms my extreme change.*

According to the doctors I will most probably never get a much lower IgE figure as they say the disease is still inside of me, but sleeping. However Reg has promised me that we are going to prove them wrong. So the next step on my journey is to build up my immune system again, and to get an IgE within the norm.

Dearest Reg, you have become a very important piece in my life, and a dear friend. I will be forever grateful for what you have done for me and look forward to continue working with you.

—Irene T. Kristensen

Before	After

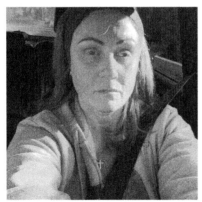 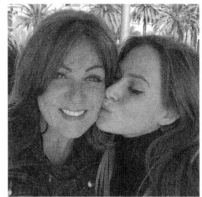

Before Her Program with Reg   *After Only 3.5 Months Of Working with Reg*

UPDATE: Two more visits to her doctor and Irene has been cleared and taken off all the drugs and medication therapy, after 30 years of being on the drugs the "Specialists" said she would be on for the rest of her life. She is a powerful lady living the life she always wanted to, free of medical limitations. "I am so proud of you Irene!! You are a true inspiration!"

bodies that keeps us healthy and disease-free. It's a crucial part of your internal environment, and the strength of your immune system relies on your choices.

Few systems in nature are as complicated as the human immune system. It exists apart from yet works in concert with every other system in the body. When it works, people stay healthy. When it malfunctions, terrible things happen. Just ask anyone who is constantly catching the latest cold going around or 'dealing with' an autoimmune disease like lupus, rheumatoid arthritis, or celiac disease.

I have personally helped hundreds of clients eliminate these horrible symptoms, some who had suffered terrible autoimmune diseases for over 30 years in some cases. One particular client was told by all the "specialists" that she would suffer from her disease for the rest of her life and eventually die from it. She was on a massive amount of medications and in terrible pain. She saw an amazing change in only three months of working with me and following the system outlined in this book. An immune system that doesn't work properly can totally upend every aspect of your life. That's why it's so important to be aware and to empower your immune system—it truly is the key to your ongoing health.

When you're able to holistically restore the flow of lymph, you're supporting immune function.

The main component of the immune system is the lymphatic system. Many people are familiar with the circulatory system, which moves blood around the body but they may not be as familiar with the lymphatic system because it isn't quite as flashy. However, the lymphatic system is extremely important. Lymph performs many vital functions in the body, especially in the context of the immune system. You have probably seen your own lymph. If you have had a cut and it ever oozed a clear fluid, that was lymph.

Lymph is initially part of the blood, but as blood flows through the body, lymph slowly leaks out. As it leaks it takes hazardous substances with it, which are filtered through the lymph nodes and trapped so they can be eliminated. Over time, the lymph steadily works its way around the body, eventually re-entering the heart so that it can be circulated all over again.

Lymph can be found all over the body, in the spaces between muscles, organs, and other structures in the body. It circulates through a series of valves, which allow the lymph to flow only in one direction. Unlike the blood, lymph does not have a central pump. It relies instead on muscle contractions and other natural functions of the body to force lymph through the lymphatic system, where it will eventually drain into the thoracic duct bringing lymph back to the heart.

Lymph fluid contains white blood cells like lymphocytes, as well as waste products and even bacteria. It circulates throughout the body, helping to fight infections. Small organs called lymph nodes are important components of the lymphatic system. These nodes are located most prominently in the throat, armpit, and groin. Lymphocytes enter the lymph nodes, where they multiply and mature, producing compounds that help fight infections. You may notice as well that your lymph nodes become swollen when you are sick because your body is isolating and making more of the agent responsible for helping you get better.

White blood cells such as lymphocytes are the main fighting soldiers in the body's immune system. They destroy foreign or diseased cells to clear them from the body. Therefore, a raised white blood cell count is often an indication of infection—the worse the infection, the more white blood cells the body sends out to fight it. That's why if you're not feeling well but there are no obvious signs of illness like an irritated throat or a runny nose, your doctor may order bloodwork.

B cells and T cells are the two main types of lymphocytes that attack foreign cells and viruses. B cells produce antibodies tailored to different cells at the command of the T cells, the regulators of the body's immune response. Those antibodies attach to foreign invaders like bacteria and viruses, either making it impossible for them to invade further, or signaling other white blood cells to come in and destroy the intruder. T cells also destroy diseased cells.

White and red blood cells are produced in the spongy tissue called bone marrow, located in the middle of your bones. That's why bone marrow is crucial for a properly functioning immune system. Leukemia, the cancer of the bone marrow, causes greatly increased production of abnormal white blood cells, and allows immature red blood cells to be released into the body. Patients who are sick with leukemia or other diseases or disorders of the immune system sometimes are told they require a bone marrow transplant to help bring back normal immune function.

Damage or interruption to the lymphatic system can result in a range of medical conditions. You may be familiar with lymphedema, a condition in which lymph pools in the limbs because it cannot circulate. Lymphoma is similarly related to the lymphatic system, as the name implies, and elephantiasis is also linked with disruption to the lymphatic system.

Lymphatic Drainage: Holistic Immune Support

Lymphatic drainage is a holistic approach to promoting a healthy lymphatic system. Although fluid moves through the lymphatic system, it does not have its own pumping mechanism. Lymph can become stagnant or slow-flowing, which can impede the normal function of your immune system. When you're able to holistically restore the flow of lymph, you're supporting immune function.

> **Unfortunately, our immune systems can also act inappropriately.**

When the lymphatic system becomes blocked, lymph nodes may become swollen. Furthermore, the system fails to remove the body's toxins and can even affect white blood cell counts. Lymphatic drainage is believed to reduce blockages that promote health in the lymphatic system, as well as other bodily systems such as the circulatory, respiratory, muscular, and endocrine systems. Lymphatic drainage therapy can also reduce allergies, menstrual cramps, colds, and other viral infections.

Lymphatic drainage is a type of therapy that is intended to help the body produce a free-flowing lymphatic system. This therapy consists of a manual massage performed by a lymphatic drainage therapist. A lymphatic drainage massage primarily focuses on specific lymph nodes and points of the body, as well as the natural flow of the lymphatic system. Proponents of lymphatic drainage believe that the process reduces blockages of the lymphatic system, which in turn promotes a healthier body. While lymphatic drainage is about preventative health care and is considered safe, physical symptoms, such as swollen lymph nodes, can indicate a problem with the lymphatic system and should be evaluated by a physician.

In addition to lymphatic drainage therapy, there is research that indicates there are additional measures people can take to promote a free-flowing lymphatic system. Some of these measures include things as simple as avoiding tight-fitting undergarments such as bras, underwear, and pantyhose, and other restrictive clothing. Tight elastic in regions where there are many lymph nodes, like the armpits and groin, can hinder the flow of lymph. Reducing stress can also help promote a healthy lymphatic system, as can regular exercise, walking at a fast pace, a healthy diet, and systematically detoxing your body.

Diseases and the Immune System

Many diseases that plague humanity are a result of insufficient immunity or an inappropriate immune response. A cold, for instance, is caused by a virus. The body doesn't immediately recognize a new virus as being harmful, so the T cell's response is, "Pass, friend," and the sneezing begins. Over time, your B cells recognize that the cold virus needs to be attacked, and they produce antibodies to help your immune system conquer that cold.

Unfortunately, our immune systems can also act inappropriately. Allergies are an example of inappropriate immune response. The body is hyper-vigilant, seeing pollen as a dangerous invader instead of a harmless yellow powder. Other diseases, such as diabetes and AIDS, suppress the immune system and reduce the body's ability to fight infection.

A great way of combating infection and illness is to go through and implement my 10 Keys.

Some vaccines are vital in helping the body fend off certain diseases, but again, in this modern world, we are seeing many examples of this going terribly wrong. As humans, we often believe that if a little works, more is better. In the olden days, a vaccine was a wise choice. The body was injected with a weakened or dead form of the virus or bacteria so it could produce the appropriate antibodies, giving complete protection against the full-strength form of the disease. This is the reason disorders such as Polio, diphtheria, mumps, and tetanus are so rarely seen today.

The problem is that vaccines have gone from a few things to support the body to a crazy concoction of hundreds of things mixed together, including actual poison, heavy metals, and other chemicals that would normally have 'danger' signs all over them, and are proven to cause way more harm than good. The intent was supposed to be that children would be vaccinated, putting the immune system on the alert. The fact is that all the stuff in the modern-day vaccines is lowering the immune response and creating all sorts of other mental and physical ailments. This is very similar to our earlier discussion regarding fire retardants and other common chemicals. They started out as a great idea, until big business and big money got involved. Now, well, we can see the results all around us, no matter what the 'specialists' and media keep telling us.

> Educate yourself first and experience how much you can enjoy conversations with the "specialists." It goes from scary and confusing to enjoyable and empowering.

Similarly, antibiotics were also designed to help the body fight disease as well. But, doctors are more cautious about prescribing broad-spectrum antibiotics since certain bacteria are starting to show resistance to them due to misuse and misunderstandings. Although antibiotics have their place, they also have the potential to do more harm than good.

Support Your Immune System Naturally

The next time you hug a loved one or smell a rose, thank your immune system. Although it can be used to fight infection, many medicines and drugs, poor nutrition, bad environments, toxic overloads, stress, lack of sleep and other issues can weaken the body's defense system. You should always consult a doctor before taking any medication. But, you also need to use common sense, be 'body wise,' and educate yourself about your life choices and what you are putting your body and mind through long before consulting any kind of "specialist." Educate yourself first and experience how much you can enjoy conversations with the "specialists." It goes from scary and confusing to enjoyable and empowering.

IMMUNITY AND THE 10 KEYS

A great way of combating infection and illness is to go through and implement my 10 Keys. Here's how the 10 Keys apply to keeping a healthy immune system:

1. Check in and ask yourself what is important to you and the impact your beliefs have on your life. Do you have any beliefs that could be affecting your immunity, like believing it's necessary to use household products that negatively impact your immune system?

2. Assess how your life and the choices you make might be affecting your immune system.

3. Tune into your body and its needs. Live mindfully and listen to your body's natural wisdom. It can be a guidance system that will help you combat any illness or ailment that keeps you from feeling your best.

4. Keep your stress levels low, get plenty of sleep, and get outside often, away from cities and electronics, to enjoy and connect with nature's medicine.

5. Pay attention to your internal and external environments. Are the things that surround you, from air quality and relationship choices to the foods and other substances you put in and on you, affecting your immune system?

6. Fuel your body with the right kind and the right amount of natural nutrients, and consistently drink pure water all day, every day.

7. Detoxify by exercising, eating whole foods, and following cleansing programs that help the body flush out harmful toxins.

8. Along with being aware and being consistently active all day, every day, make sure you schedule 'you time' at least 30 minutes a day, every day. Movement helps keep the immune system healthy, even simple things like regularly walking, dancing, gardening; anything that moves your body. Exercise also boosts the circulatory system, naturally helping your body detox, and it reduces the risk of certain diseases. Exercise does not have to be a workout in the gym.

9. Put support systems in place to reinforce the small changes you are implementing to become the best version of you.

10. Be aware of the choices you are making and who you are sharing you with.

> ## When you're diagnosed with something, how do you avoid the fear and pressure to do "whatever" forced on you by the "specialists" and your family and friends?

Here are some other lifestyle tips to help you support your immune system naturally:

FOOD AND YOUR IMMUNE SYSTEM

It's important to note here that one of the major threats to the immune system is the lifestyle choice known as eating. Consuming pre-packaged, pre-made, processed, and fast foods, along with all the added and extra 'sugary treats' every day, is even worse than smoking. Yup, I said it. Smoking is horrible for your body for countless reasons. Many smokers find themselves with constant colds and viral infections. Smoking seriously harms and weakens the immune system. But, when you're not fueling your body the way it needs with the fuel it requires, recognizes, and actually uses, you are on a fast trip to bad health and endless negative issues. The next time you are in a busy public place, stop for a moment and just watch people. Really look at them: their skin, their eyes, the shape of their bodies, and how they move. I know people who have been smoking for 80 years or more, and who still seem to be pretty healthy and active. I know people who have been eating crap food for 20 or 30 years who are in way worse condition than the smokers. But, when you combine the two, well, it's a losing combination and it's a fast track to the afterworld, after a whole lot of suffering first.

You need to eat plenty of real, live, natural, fresh foods, fruit and vegetables every day to keep your body in top shape. Eating pre-made, processed, and fast foods only slows the mind's functionality, the body's immune system, and your metabolism. Natural and fresh foods are rich in vitamins and minerals and help keep the immune system powerful. Older people and pregnant women will especially benefit from eating clean, natural foods that are rich in essential nutrients.

If you are bringing a child into this world, you should be even more aware of your choices, as everything you do will affect that child's entire life, and the lives of their children, too. My number one suggestion to all parents and parents-to-be is to become aware! Really think about what you are feeding yourself and your children, and what these choices are doing to you and your children, their entire lives, and in turn, their children.

> If you are bringing a child into this world, you should be even more aware of your choices, as everything you do will affect that child's entire life, and the lives of their children, too.

If you are now pregnant, be aware! Everything about you will affect your child. Everything from the foods you eat to your moods, your activity levels, your environment, the products you use, and the water you wash them in, together with your choices and your beliefs all go directly into that child. Your child will live with all that for their entire life, and then pass it on to their children. If you at some point want to have children, be aware! You and the partner you choose will together create a mix of you both that will go into creating this brand-new life. If you have ever wondered why so many children these days are being born with all these terrible health issues, simple look at the parents, their environments, their relationships, their choices of foods, the products they use every day, and their life choices and it becomes very clear.

If you already have children, be aware! Stop believing you are doing them or you a favor, saving time or money, or being 'nice' by giving them 'sugary treats', dairy, wheat, processed, pre-made, and fast foods. You are NOT being nice and these things are NOT 'treats.' In fact, those beliefs and choices are ensuring that you, your children, and your grandchildren will have endless ailments and issues to deal with. These issues will drastically affect their moods, concentration, growth, mental state, education, career, relationships, family dynamics, success and every other aspect of their lives, and in turn affect your life and the lives of your friends and family around you. All around us, it's easy to see the endless list of ailments and illnesses that are driven by your beliefs, the choices you make every minute of every day, the stuff you're putting in and on your body, the people you share your energy with, and your home environment. All you need to do is open your eyes and be aware. If you or your children are dealing with or suffering from hyperactivity, ADHD, or any other label, ailment, or illness, then the first things to look at are your beliefs that may be causing you to choose what goes in, on, and around your body, and ask yourself whether those beliefs could be contributing to the creation these negative situations.

> **Different people need varying amounts of sleep, depending on your lifestyle and natural energy burn, but enforcing eight hours per night should be at the top of your "Must-Do" list.**

Cutting out foods and drinks with high caffeine content is also a good idea. You'll be your best natural self when you get your energy from whole, natural foods, not artificially from chemically-enhanced, energetically-dead foods and beverages. Drinking plenty of pure, clean water helps flush harmful toxins from the body. Natural, pure, fresh fruit juices also provide countless benefits, and there are plenty of herbal teas that can be a great substitute for regular tea and coffee.

GET ENOUGH SLEEP

The amount of high-quality sleep you get nightly in a healthy environment is a vital factor in keeping the immune system health. This absolutely cannot be ignored or belittled. Ensuring you are breathing in clean, fresh air during your sleep cycle encourages and supports the body to repair itself and to remain fighting fit and naturally energized. Sleep is also a great stress reducer, and getting enough sleep helps lower your cortisol levels. When the body is stressed, it produces more cortisol, which weakens both your immune system and your mind.

Different people need varying amounts of sleep, depending on your lifestyle and natural energy burn, but enforcing eight hours per night should be at the top of your "Must-Do" list. The key here is to be aware of you and your body. This is not the time to be "the tough guy" or to prove to the world your superpowers which allow you to drink coffee and supercharged drinks, eat super processed and magical 'foods' created in a lab, and only sleep between phone calls or while waiting for the red light. Don't fool yourself due to your beliefs and ego; your body and mind MUST sleep.

> Don't fool yourself due to your beliefs and ego; your body and mind MUST sleep.

Believing you can get away with only a few hours a night, or whatever you can fit it in, will absolutely drastically affect how your body and mind function, and it will significantly affect your long-term health and performance levels, too. There are countless medical, university, and real-life tests that have proven this, yet I still see individuals claiming to only sleep two to four hours and they are 'doing just great!' Sure, they're doing great until 'all of a sudden' they are not doing so great anymore. Lying to yourself and believing you can cheat the body to accomplish more is just as bad, if not worse, then all the other things we have and will cover in this book. Just like smoking, eating bad foods, drugs, bad relationships, and all the other things affecting your long-term health, it may seem you can go without much sleep with no issues now, but you can be sure things will not always be like they are right now, and often times things radically change, really, really fast.

Your immune system is always patrolling, always on guard, and always ready to go on Red Alert until the day you die. It's patrolling and guarding while you're awake, while you're asleep, while you are moving about, and while you are at rest. It's important to take extremely good care of your immune system for it to take the best care of you. Your immunity is your key to a joyful, productive, accomplished, and long life. This is the meaning of the often-used phrase, "If you have your health, you have everything."

> People who are highly effective, accomplished, and successful know that they must do everything they can to maintain a healthy immune system *first and always.*

People who are highly effective, accomplished, and successful know that they must do everything they can to maintain a healthy immune system *first and always.* The internal system is designed to support the best version of you, and it's not something to ignore.

Key Takeaways:

You must support the health of your immune system if you want live the life you love and love the life you live, long term.

Your lymphatic system is a vital part of your immune system and your internal environment.

Lymphatic drainage therapy can help you support the health of your immune system naturally by keeping lymph and white blood cells moving through your body freely, supporting the flow to naturally eliminate inflammation, pain and disease.

Be aware! Support your immune system naturally by paying close attention to what you put in and on your body, and in and on the bodies of your children. Stop smoking, eat lots of fruits and vegetables, and reduce or eliminate sugar and caffeine.

Make sure you're getting a minimum of eight hours sleep every night. Sleep is crucial to keep your mind and your immune system healthy and happy.

"

Let food be thy medicine
and medicine be thy food.

—HIPPOCRATES

Eating for Your Healthiest Self

There's a reason why the saying, "You are what you eat," gets repeated over and over again. The food you choose to fuel your body with has a huge impact on your health, your mood, and your overall wellbeing. There is a massive difference between filling your stomach and fueling your body. When people think about getting healthy, they often immediately think of hitting the gym or dieting. But, often dieting becomes more about depriving yourself of certain foods than about properly fueling your body.

> Fueling your body with the right food will help you and your family develop and maintain great health for many, many years to come, while enriching and empowering all the other aspects of your life.

The Natural You approach focuses on the quality and quantity of the foods you eat. If you remember from earlier in the book, it's essential that you get the right macro- and micronutrients from your food if you're going to achieve optimal health. This chapter will serve as a guide to help you understand how you can use food and supplements to ensure great health, high levels of natural energy, a clear mind, healthy skin, hair, eyes, and organs, and to heal yourself naturally. Fueling your body with the right food will help you and your family develop and maintain great health for many, many years to come, while enriching and empowering all the other aspects of your life.

Sugar: Hero or Villain?

Refined sugar is one of the biggest causes of health harms in our modern society. It is the most overlooked item we consume in terms of the impact on our internal and external environment. Many of us, including most of our children, are completely addicted to sugar. When you eat sugar, your brain releases many of the same chemicals that are released when you take an opioid drug or heroin.[1] In fact, according to medical science, sugar is eight times more addictive then cocaine or heroin. That, combined with its negative effects on your health, makes sugar one of the most dangerous and influential substances you consume on a regular basis.

> **Refined sugar is one of the biggest causes of health harms in our modern society.**

In this section, I will examine the different types of sugar, where they come from, and how to eliminate the unnecessary sugar from your life. I will prove to you that probably no other food on our table is as controversial and so dangerous as refined sugar, and how detrimental it is to your internal and external environment, and to the developing minds and bodies of our children.

All carbohydrates are composed of simple or complex sugar molecules. These include:

- The monosaccharides such as glucose and fructose, which are constructed from a single sugar molecule and are incapable of being broken down further during digestion.

---

[1] Avena, N. M., Rada, P., & Hoebel, B. G. (2008). Evidence for sugar addiction: behavioral and neurochemical effects of intermittent, excessive sugar intake. *Neuroscience & biobehavioral reviews*, 32(1), 20-39

- The disaccharides, or double sugars—like sucrose (table sugar) and lactose—which are made of two monosaccharides.

- The polysaccharides, such as starch and fiber, which are composed of two or more simple sugars that are less water soluble, more stable, and slower to break down in the intestines.

These compounds are necessary for your body's sustenance and welfare. Without them, you perish. And all of them are sugars.

> I will prove to you that probably no other food on our table is as controversial and so dangerous as refined sugar, and how detrimental it is to your internal and external environment, and to the developing minds and bodies of our children.

However, refined sugar is not your friend. It may make you feel good when you hang out together, but the pleasure doesn't last. Have you ever paid attention to how your body feels or to your mood after indulging in sugar? Sure, you might feel great right after you eat it, but then the crash happens. Your energy is low, you may be more irritable than usual, and your cravings for more sugary treats are stronger.

Here's why: sugar is not a real food. Food can be described as any substance that provides nourishment for the human body. The components of nourishment are protein, fats, complex carbohydrates, vitamins, and minerals. When you consume sugar, your body isn't getting any of these—no nourishment at all—NONE! Usually it's just your mind creating nurturing thoughts like, "Ooh, delicious," and, "This is so yummy," or, "now I have the energy to do what I need to do," which leads to you believing you are satisfied. I have some bad news: that's a fantasy, and what your body is really saying is, "Hey, I need some nourishment! Please, I am losing energy. I don't think I can digest this food properly and I am going to need to store it." Believe me, I love sweets too, so I am not saying go out and deprive yourself. All I am

THE DANGERS OF SUGAR

Today, the majority of people who eat a 'normal western diet' are completely and totally addicted to sugar.

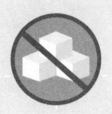

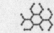

HYPERTENSION

CARDIOVASCULAR DISEASE

HYPOGLYCEMIA

ADD/ADHD

METABOLIC SYNDROME

DIZZINESS

OBESITY

ALLERGIES

TOOTH DECAY

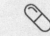

CHOLESTEROL

COLON & PANCREATIC CANCER

TYPE 2 DIABETES

suggesting is that you should be more aware about how sugar impacts your health. And, if you must have it, use it as a small addition once in a while rather than the one thing you use and take in every time you put something in your mouth.

The following list is based on data issued by the USDA and shows the nutrients present in table sugar (sucrose):[2]

NUTRIENTS	AMOUNT (MG)	NUTRIENTS	AMOUNT (MG)
Protein	0	Thiamine	0
Fats	0	Riboflavin	0
Vitamin A	0	Calcium	0
Vitamin C	0	Iron	0
Vitamin D	0	Sodium	.24
Vitamin E	0	Potassium	.76
Niacin	0	Phosphorus	0

The sum of nutrients in sugar is a good deal less than one milligram per ounce. One milligram is a thousandth of a gram, and there are just over 28 grams in an ounce. The sodium and potassium present in sugar are in the form of a salt, but again, there is more potassium in the paper on this page than in an ounce of sugar.

Refined sugar is sugar cane that has been denatured, heated, filtered, rubbed, evaporated, and clarified, had its color—and all the natural, healthy elements it naturally has—removed, and then adulterated with lime and diatomaceous earth. All the cane's natural nutrients are removed, and the leftovers are bottled and sold as molasses.

No, you are getting to know my mentality a bit more, so I must ask the question: why are we eating so much sugar? Why go through all that work to change what nature naturally provides as healthy, useful, great tasting, and highly beneficial, and why change it to something that creates so much harm to the body and mind? And then, why is it

[2] United States Department of Agriculture. (2016). *Food Composition Databases Show Foods— Sugars, granulated.* Retrieved from https://ndb.nal.usda.gov/ndb/foods/show/6319.

intentionally put it into almost every processed food, drink, and "health food" available in the stores today? *Why?* Why not just use the natural stuff? Why do we allow big business to do this with every natural food and product on earth? Besides big business money making even more money, I will never understand this. More than not understanding this, I am even more confused as to why everyone living on this planet supports, encourages, and allows this to happen. I feel this is very strange, from my own imperfect perception.

> ## All I am suggesting is that you should be more aware about how sugar impacts your health.

In the book *Diet for a Small Planet*, Frances Moore Lappé took a good, hard look at the composition of foodstuffs based on a government handbook. Ms. Lappé reported that 3.5 ounces of sugar lacked most vitamins or minerals, containing only 1 mg of sodium and 3 mg of potassium. Conversely, the same amount of molasses contained over 2.9 g of potassium (975 times more than sugar) and 96 mg of sodium (which is, of course, 96 times the sodium found in sugar). Molasses also contained 684 mg of calcium, 84 mg phosphorous, 16 mg of iron, 0.19 mg of vitamin B2, 0.11 mg of vitamin B1, and 0.2 mg of vitamin B3, which were all undetectable in the table sugar.[3]

Not only is sugar almost completely void of micronutrients, but it's also difficult for your body to digest. When sugar reaches your digestive tract, it needs a certain number of vitamins and minerals to be metabolized, plus small amounts of protein and fat. As it burns up these vital materials, it fails to replace them with equivalent energies. It uses more energy to consume than it provides.

After excessive sugar consumption, so many vitamins and minerals get removed and depleted from the cells that the body begins to weaken. All the excess sugar that pours into your body can no longer be burned away. So, that extra sugar is transformed into fatty adipose tissue. It gets stored away, adding to your waistline and harming your health. This means that throughout your journey of gaining weight, becoming obese will not only

---

[3] Lappé, F. M. (2011). *Diet for a Small Planet: The Book That Started a Revolution in the Way Americans Eat.* Ballantine Books.

make your body larger, and make all your systems have to work harder, but at the same time your body is becoming more and more malnourished.

This is also why many overweight people claim, "I'm always hungry, even after eating." Well, you're still hungry because when you eat crap food—food that's pre-packaged, pre-made, processed, fast 'food,' and all those sugary 'treats'—you're not feeding your body! All you have done is feed the cravings of your mind, and your body is still waiting for something it can use as fuel. Your body needs you to be ingesting natural foods that your body can actually use. It may taste great, but it's like putting water in the tank of your car. The gas gauge shows full, but the engine is starving. Worse yet, sugar causes inflammation in your body[4], which leaves you susceptible to a large range of diseases, from autoimmune disorders to cancer, and so much more.

> It may taste great, but it's like putting water in the tank of your car.

CAN YOU AVOID SUGAR?

If sugar's so bad for you, all you have to do is avoid eating it, right? Unfortunately, that's easier said than done. Sugar is hidden in almost every processed food you eat. It's harder and harder to avoid due to big business continually coming up with new names for the stuff.

So again, I ask, why? If we live in a world that is run by governments and businesses that state they want us to be healthy, happy people, knowing what we know about the effects that this one product has on the human body, why is it not only allowed to *be in* but also to be *hidden in* almost everything we eat?

Here's a fun challenge: see how many pre-packaged and processed items you can find that do *not* contain added sugars. Here's a partial list of items in which sucrose is found: nearly all canned soups, fruits and vegetables, beer, wine, liquor, bread, mayonnaise, non-dairy cream, salt, some smoked foods, olives, certain cheeses, artificial sweeteners, hot dogs, peanut butter, baby food, canned clams, ketchup, mustard,

---

[4] Aeberli, I., Gerber, P. A., Hochuli, M., Kohler, S., Haile, S. R., Gouni-Berthold, I., ... & Berneis, K. (2011). Low to moderate sugar-sweetened beverage consumption impairs glucose and lipid metabolism and promotes inflammation in healthy young men: a randomized controlled trial. *The American journal of clinical nutrition*, 94(2), 479-485.

Reg's Natural You Tweaks

1. **Check the labels on the foods in your pantry.** Look on the side of the bottle or package and start to notice what kinds of sugars are being used in the products you eat on a regular basis. Be aware that manufacturers often substitute the term "sucrose," "corn syrup," or "pure cane sugar" for alternative sugar names in the hope that you'll think it's a healthy derivative or something other than what it really is.

2. **Drop sugar—all sugar—from your diet for two weeks and begin to journal about your journey.** See how you feel after only 24 hours without it. Start now, today, immediately. Next meal, leave the sugar out of your coffee or tea. Forget the fake sweet dessert and have fun creating your own naturally sweet and tasty treats. The internet is packed with endless powerful and delicious ideas. My suggestion is that you work towards cutting *all* processed foods out of your life. It really is not so hard or time consuming as you may believe right now. Once you get into it and make it your own, you will wonder why you were ever eating the old way. Any fast food place has sugar in pretty much everything. Avoid all pre-made and fast foods and see how you feel. Please note: if you try thinking of sneaky ways to "accidentally" sneak sugar into the two weeks, you are addicted! Cravings usually indicate that your body has a physical and psychological addiction to sugar. Be aware that when you cut sugar out of your diet, you will go through withdrawal symptoms, just like any other drug addict. You could experience headaches, body aches, fever, and many, many other symptoms. But that just goes to prove how addicted your body is to this stuff.

3. **Dedicate yourself to one full week of absolutely no sugar and experience how coming off it affects every aspect of your life.** Go through the challenges and discomfort with an open mind, willing to clearly understand and experience your body as the amazing body it is. Give it time to eliminate all that stuff it has been wanting to clear out for a very long time, and allow yourself to learn and truly understand how something this small can impact your body, health, relationships, work, and life so much.

bouillon cubes, tomato sauce, pickles, pancake mix, most breakfast cereals, virtually all frozen ready meals, all cured foods, jams and jellies, cigarettes, pasta, vitamins, salad dressing, almost all fast foods like salads, pizza, burgers, and chicken.

Today, the majority of people who eat a 'normal western diet' are completely and totally addicted to sugar. Of course, in this modern world we live in, when we discover a food product is harmful to us, we should then create a "substitute" or healthier option. But do we? Is the 'health food' you pay a lot more money for actually healthier?

THE DANGERS OF SUGAR SUBSTITUTES

We are generally becoming more aware and educated, and we do understand that sugar is bad. So, what do the modern big businesses do? Do they eliminate it to help us become healthier? No. They say, "Here, eat this sugar substitute called saccharin (which is derived from coal tar)," or countless other options with strange names created in science labs and filled with even worse stuff creating even more harm to your body. Many of these "healthy" ingredients are the same substances used to make insect repellent, perfumes, and creosote, yet it is legal to put in your food, and it's approved and protected by big government and the FDA.

Here's an example. Saccharin was discovered approximately a century ago and was promptly removed from consumption when its harmful properties were recognized. It oddly returned to the marketplace of our wise modern world because Teddy Roosevelt was on a diet and found it to be his ideal alternative to sugar. Even though saccharin has long been linked to cancer and is banned in a few countries, including several in the former Soviet Union, it has remained in production ever since. Insanity at its finest, don't you think? Or, is there more to it?

Tests in Canada in the 1970s demonstrated that people who eat saccharin are twice as likely to develop cancer as those who don't. Pregnant women and very young children should avoid it entirely. Many studies indicate that both the fetus and the newborn are particularly vulnerable to its effects.[5] Here is another question: why is it normal to read "If you're pregnant avoid this . . ." but if you're not pregnant it's

---

[5] Cohen-Addad, N., Chatterjee, M., Bekersky, I., & Blumenthal, H. P. (1986). In utero-exposure to saccharin: a threat? *Cancer letters*, 32(2), 151-154.

okay to eat it? Shouldn't something that harms your body or a child in your body be avoided all the time?

> Dedicate yourself to one full week of absolutely no sugar and experience how coming off it affects every aspect of your life.

BENEFITS OF ELIMINATING SUGAR

Sugar's impact on your internal environment can cause a spectrum of health problems, from cravings because your body feels deprived of nourishment, to diabetes and cancer because of the inflammation sugar creates in the body. Cutting out sugar completely may feel too challenging—I get it. We live in a world addicted to it, and big business puts it in pretty much everything, so yes, it is challenging, but only at first.

If you truly want to reduce the amount of sugar you eat, focus on all the benefits eliminating sugar could offer you. Here are some: you gain a more consistent powerful mind and mental clarity, decrease your body fat, improve the health of your skin, teeth, eyes and organs, and cultivate natural endurance because your body is being properly nourished from the inside out. When you nourish your body with stuff it is naturally designed to use, your natural energy levels go way up. You find you sleep better, have better concentration, your headaches and body aches will decrease or go away altogether, your mood will be more balanced, and you'll get to enjoy all the amazing natural flavors you have been missing out on, all while living a much more enjoyable life. Are all these natural and free benefits worth trying new things and learning new habits for? Only you can make that choice.

It is worth starting today. Start small and be aware of everything you eat and drink. Before buying it or eating it, just ask yourself: is this adding to better health, happiness, and success of my body and mind, and those of my family, or taking me away from it? Every time you make a choice to avoid eating or drinking sugar is a WIN for better health and a better life. You don't want to lose being on top of your game because you are losing a battle with one of the biggest villains we face in relation to our health, happiness, and success today. Or, you could simply ask yourself: what's more important? That sugary treat and processed food, or your long-term health, happiness, and success?

> Are all these natural and free benefits worth trying new things and learning new habits for? Only you can make that choice.

Supplement Your Health and Wellness

Earlier in the book we discussed our internal environments, and I mentioned the environmental elements our body needs. These components act as nutrients. Our body and mind need clarity and awareness, motivated actions, positive choices, people who empower us and hold us accountable to better lifestyle choices, careers that inspire us, and homes that are supportive, relaxing, empowering, fun, and free from toxins. Another way to provide nutrients to your internal environment is through supplements.

For most of us today, a healthy diet and lifestyle isn't enough to provide us with the full scope and range of nutrients that we need. Food just isn't what it used to be. We are not eating the same fruit, veggies, meat, and dairy that our grandparents ate; everything has changed. Supplements can be a simple solution with huge benefits. As I mentioned at the beginning of the book, my goal is to outline simple steps that will support you to be the best, most natural version of you.

Adding pure, natural supplements will support you in:
- Sustaining a strong immune system,
- Reducing your need for pharmaceuticals,
- Maintaining your health and wellness goals,
- Maintaining your natural healthy weight,
- Enhancing your clear and powerful mind, and
- Ensuring your body is being fueled rather than filled, so the blood, organs, muscles, and other systems receive all they need in order to ensure your body and mind are all performing at ultimate levels of production and efficiency.

In this section, I will help you learn how to avoid some of the problems with selecting products, how to understand what your body may be lacking, which supplements specifically to focus on, and where to find the products that can help you achieve the quality of life you've always dreamed of.

Today's market is exploding with health and fitness supplements as more people realize their efficacy and the needs that they fulfill. The plethora of health and wellness supplement products on the market is overwhelming, so how do you select the right ones? With so many similar products by different manufacturers to choose from, all making competing claims of quality and effectiveness, how do you know which to spend your money on? Should you learn by trial and error? Should you wade through the sea of articles, blogs, and product reviews hoping to get your answers?

Let's make your search smarter, not harder. When you fuel your body with natural products, your body absorbs all or most of the nutrients contained in the supplement, rather than storing it in your body or flushing it down the toilet. There are a few smart things you can do quickly, like taking the most suitable dietary supplements around. The following are supplements I recommend adding into your life immediately:

Take a probiotic. The secret to good health, both mental and physical, lies in the friendly bacteria in the intestinal tract. *Lactobacillus* bacteria form a significant part of the natural intestinal flora. Large populations of these and other lactic acid-producing bacteria regulate the levels of friendly bacteria, reduce the levels of toxic pathogens that cause ill health, and even affect the levels of neurotransmitters in your body that regulate your mood. The ability of the bacteria in the gut to thrive is the single most important factor in a probiotic product. The bacteria must be in their natural state and alive (therefore, only buy probiotics stored in a refrigerated case) so that once they arrive in the gut they can multiply and produce all the sub-strains necessary to maintain a healthy intestinal flora.

Take a strong enzyme. Enzymes, in general, help deliver nutrients, carry away toxic waste, digest food, purify the blood, deliver hormones by feeding and fortifying the endocrine system, balance cholesterol and triglyceride levels, feed the brain, and cause no harm to the body. These factors all contribute to the strengthening of the immune system, as well as strengthening your overall health.

Take cat's claw. Cat's claw is derived from an Amazonian vine, and it works to support your immunity naturally, as well as acting as an anti-inflammatory and antioxidant. When using a powdered extract, taking 1 to 3 500mg capsules up to 3 to 4 times daily may be sufficient to alleviate many health problems. If you can find it in liquid form, even better.

Take MSM. The health benefits of MSM *(methyl-sulfonyl-methane)* are vast and as such it has become a very popular natural treatment for arthritis and related ailments. MSM is a natural sulfur compound found in the oceans, rainwater, and all living things, including you. Sulfurous amino acids protect us against the effects of radiation and heavy metals. Methionine helps draw heavy metals out of the body, and is found in high concentrations in raw pumpkin seeds. Cystine and cysteine, found in hemp seeds, are almost identical. Cysteine is present in hair, keratin, and insulin, and it helps make your skin more flexible. It also supports your body's natural collagen, not only keeping you looking younger, but also helping to protect tissues from damage.

I take two tablespoons of pure organic MSM powder daily. Every day, my first morning and last evening drink is a big bottle of pure ionized water. I squeeze in one big fresh lemon, and add in one tablespoon of pure MSM, one tablespoon of pure organic Vitamin C powder, and sometimes I'll add in some pure raw mint or cinnamon, a little pure organic local honey, and a pinch of pink Himalayan sea salt. I drink two of these bottles every day. All of these ingredients readily available online or in a good health food store. Try it for four weeks and see if you notice any changes in your body and mind.

Taking Your Vitamins

There are a few vitamins that you should also take regularly because they can help you live a naturally healthier life. I personally recommend (and take) both a vitamin C and vitamin D supplement. Many of us are chronically low on these two important vitamins, and when we add high-quality vitamin C and D supplements to our diets, our internal environments are dramatically improved.

VITAMIN C

Vitamin C, also known as ascorbic acid, is a water-soluble vitamin which is essential for normal functioning of the body. Vitamin C is an antioxidant, and it also acts as a cofactor, helping several enzymes present in our cells function properly. Because it is an essential nutrient, our bodies

Reg's Natural You Tweaks

1. Get customized. In some ways your body is just like everyone else's, yet at the same time it is totally unique, as are your lifestyle and your beliefs. You need supplements that are better suited for *your* body's specific wants and needs. Remember, if you're tested and find you are low on nutrients but you claim you "eat a lot" of them, then a broader look is required.

Before dumping more money into more products, detox first. A huge majority of the clients I work with eliminate many of their ailments and issues by detoxing first. Remember, clean first, and then add in the good stuff, just like changing the oil in a car. Find a great live blood analysis or functional medicine specialist and get tested to help assess your supplementary needs based upon where your body is now. Don't get sucked into buying more stuff, but do get very clear in exactly what you are dealing with and the potential reasons for any ailments, issues, or imbalances.

Think smart and get to know how your body functions. When you are given information, you will know what to do and why you're doing it. This is a far better way to live, rather than just trusting what everyone is telling you is fact and trying endless ways to deal with it. It may surprise you just how cheap and easy it is to empower your body and mind, to make your own products, and fulfill your body's natural needs by eating and using natural stuff. There are many websites out there that teach you how to make your own supplements. Save yourself time and money and break free from the chemical-based stuff, which is causing endless issues in all aspects of your life. Avoid the stuff that we have all been brainwashed to believe we need and are paying way too much for.

2. Find the right suppliers. Health and fitness supplements in their pure and natural form are generally the best, and there are a few really exceptional suppliers online who invest the time and put in the effort to provide top-rate supplements made from clean, organic products, void of chemical fillers and sugars. Standard pills and capsules allow too much of their nutrient quality to be passed out of the body in the metabolic process. Many of the 'natural' products that are sold in the more common shops generally use products crammed full with fillers and extras that you do not want or need.

Another important point to note is that due to endless regulations on 'natural' products, the quantity as well as the quality of the actual ingredient that you wish to be using is usually in such small dosages that the 'recommended' amounts you are to take is nowhere near correct. This is why we often hear "I took that natural stuff and it didn't do anything for me."

Do your research, get to know what you're taking, how much you need to be taking, and for how long you should be taking it for, in order to achieve your needs and save you a lot of time and money. Ensure that your health and fitness supplements are all-natural and don't contain any fillers. In fact, I almost never purchase "multi-" anything. I choose to buy all organic and natural individual products, and then I mix my own blends. This way, I get exactly what I want, and I can play with how much I take. So, while listening to my body, I get very clear on how much I need, or if I even need it any more. When you buy pre-mixed stuff, you have no clarity as to exactly what it is you are taking, and you can only trust or guess as to how much you're really actually getting.

3. What do I take regularly? Again, I believe in variety and change. Our bodies are alive, meaning they change, and what they need and what you do with them and for them also changes. There are not many products I would suggest taking regularly, however there are a few.

This is a list of good and not so good things, products habits and choices, stuff to make sure I'm using regularly, or avoiding it intentionally.

AILMENT AND ILLNESS GROWTH PROMOTERS
- Too much insulin—sugar, high glycemic diets
- Too much insulin-like growth factor (IGF-1) (e.g. dairy)
- Too much cortisol—stress, stimulants
- Excess estrogen—linked to excess body fat
- Progesterone deficiency—linked to anovulation
- Lack of estrogen blockers/phytoestrogens—beans, etc.
- Lack of estrogen detoxifiers—greens, poor liver function
- Lack of good quality sleep

- Environmental chemicals: toothpaste, laundry detergents, deodorants, hair gels and sprays, shampoos, antibacterial soaps and cleaners, skin creams, sunscreens
- Lack of sunshine
- Lack of clean air
- Drinking tap and plastic bottle water.

TOP TIPS FOR 100% IMMUNITY

1. Don't smoke and minimize pollution exposure
2. No more than one unit of alcohol a day, and preferably not every day
3. Reduce stress and get enough sleep—between 6.5 and 8 hours minimum.
4. Exercise regularly preferably in natural daylight—get outdoors
5. Eat lots of fresh fruit and vegetables
6. Eat something orange, blue, red, and dark green every day—the more natural colors you eat, the better.
7. Eat a low glycemic and low dairy diet (less red meat, more fish)
8. Don't eat foods you are allergic too, and if you are allergic, find out exactly why.
9. Have half your diet raw and avoid fried foods
10. Supplement 1-3 grams of zinc, berry extracts, and other antioxidants and immune friendly nutrients, daily—twice a day.

IMMUNE HEROES:

- Vitamin C
- Selenium
- Zinc
- B vitamins
- N-acetyl cysteine
- Vitamin D
- Essential (especially omega 3) fats
- Black elderberry (for viruses)
- Herbs—Echinacea, *Uncaria tomentosa* (cat's claw) etc.
- Beneficial bacteria (*Acidophilus* and bifidobacteria)
- Vitamin A
- Beta Carotene
- Vitamin E
- Co-Q10
- Alpha lipoic acid
- Glutathione
- Selenium
- Resveratrol
- Bilberry extract
- Ginger

SUPERFOODS

- Broccoli contains I3C and DIM which mop up excess estrogens.
- Watercress contains isothiocyanate which turns off cancer cells.
- Strawberries have more vitamin C than oranges, while blueberries have among the highest ORAC score due to their anthocyanin bioflavonoids. Strawberries and raspberries also contain ellagic acid, which help protect against cancer.
- Red onions contain quercetin, a potent anti-inflammatory.
- Carrots, and other orange foods such as sweet potato and butternut squash contain carotenoids and other anti-cancer nutrients.
- Turmeric and ginger are anti-inflammatories. Curcumin, in turmeric, has anti-cancer properties.
- Liquid flax seed oil (non-lignin)
- Pure cinnamon powder
- Raw brown or golden flax seeds
- Wheatgrass
- Chlorophyll
- Beets
- Celery
- Spinach
- Asparagus. For treatment of lots of ailments and life-threatening disease, use only organic fresh asparagus. It should be cooked before using. Source local providers who ensure it contain no pesticides or preservatives. Place the cooked asparagus in a blender and liquefy to make a puree. Store in the refrigerator. Take four full tablespoons twice daily, morning and evening.
- *Moringa oleifera* (Also known as the "Drumstick tree" or the "Horseradish tree" or the "Miracle tree")
- *Spirulina*
- Mixed greens
- Living full super greens
- Cucumber
- Apples
- Apricot kernels
- Arugula
- Hot peppers
- Garlic
- Bok choy
- Cabbage
- Cauliflower
- Chives
- Leeks
- Peas
- Onions
- Sauerkraut
- Shallots
- Avocados
- Essiac tea
- Cellect powder

OTHER KEY IMMUNE-BOOSTING NUTRIENTS

- Selenium is required for glutathione related activity and has anti-cancer properties. Found in seafood, it is frequently deficient. Aim to supplement 100mcg if compromised immunity.
- N-acetyl cysteine is the precursor of glutathione, the most critical antioxidant in cells. NAC improves the anti-viral function of vitamin C.
- B6, B12, folic acid are anti-oxidants and required for methylation. Faulty methylation is associated with increased cancer risk.
- Vitamin A, both retinol and beta-carotene, is anti-viral, stimulates T-cell growth, and makes cells strong. For example, transdermal vitamin A protects against skin cancer.
- The amino acids lysine, proline, and N-acetyl cysteine, as well as selenium. N-acetyl cysteine and selenium both promote glutathione levels within cells, which has anti-viral activity.

4. I highly recommend that you add the following products to your daily routine, and research to see why, what they actually do for you and how you feel when taking them. Plus, as you become more aware and you simplify your life and your body's needs, you can have fun while expanding your experiences to add more of your own:

- Pure, clean, organic hemp protein is the best on the market and for your body. I invite you to spend 20 minutes researching hemp and all its great benefits. I make a hemp protein shake every morning, mixed with a tablespoon of super greens, a teaspoon of organic bee pollen, a tablespoon of organic pumpkin, hemp hearts, linseeds, a shot of pure organic juice, some organic coconut oil, and a few different fruits and veggies . . . yummy! *Note: I suggest avoiding whey and soy protein powders altogether.

- Udo's 3-6-9 oil blends is, as of the time I'm writing this, my favorite. I put a tablespoon in all my shakes and on my salads.

- Pure organic vitamin C powder: put two tablespoons into each of two-liter glass bottles of pure water (four tablespoons total). Refer to the previous section about MSM for the recipe for the water I drink every day. You can heat it up or add ice to it, hot or cold, all year round. Sip on it all day until both bottles are finished. Do this every day for the next three months and watch and feel how your body changes.

If you're feeling sick, drink lots of this. And, you can add in 1 teaspoon of pure organic cayenne pepper and 10 drops of pure medical grade oil of oregano. This is a great way to kill of infection, inflammation, and disease.

don't create it on their own, which means we need to get our vitamin C from our diets. Foods that are naturally rich in vitamin C include kale, broccoli, Brussels sprouts, strawberries, citrus fruits, and kiwi fruit.

Much of what we know about the benefits for vitamin C comes from pioneering researcher Irwin Stone.[6] Stone scoured the research literature for scientific evidence that showed the important health benefits of this vitamin. In his book, *The Healing Factor: Vitamin C Against Disease*, he detailed how vitamin C can help combat everything from viral infections to allergies to diabetes. Stone's work is unique and incredibly valuable. The complete text of *The Healing Factor*, previously a hard-to-find book, is now posted for free reading at https://vitamincfoundation.org/stone.

You should strongly consider adding a high-quality vitamin C supplement to your daily routine today. Along with regularly eating a lot of proteins, carbs, fats, fresh fruit and veggies, I take MSM and vitamin C daily, starting the moment I wake up. This daily habit helps me support my immune system, and helps me function at my highest level possible mentally and physically.

VITAMIN D

Another thing I always tell my clients is to "let the sun shine in." Yes, real sunshine. Vitamin D is one of the most powerful healing chemicals in your body—your body makes it for free every day. There is no prescription required, no sales made. For those of you worried about UV exposure, I'm happy to inform you that it turns out that *super antioxidants greatly boost your body's ability to handle sunlight without burning*. Astaxanthin is one of the most powerful "internal sunscreens" and can allow you to stay in the sun twice as long without burning. The best thing to do is get outside every day, all year round, no matter where you live, and spend time every day in the sun.

What are your beliefs about the sun? Are your fears about sun exposure from real, actual human being facts? Or, are your fears just based on what you have heard? If you are an individual who easily burns in the sun, have you really researched why?

You may be just as shocked as I was when I found these statistics about vitamin D deficiency[7]:

---

[6] Saul, A.W. (2005). Irwin Stone: Orthomolecular educator and innovator. *J Orthomolecular Med.* 20(4), 230-236.

[7] Adams, M, & Holick, M. (2005, January 1). Vitamin D Myths, Facts and Statistics. Retrieved July 11, 2017 from http://www.naturalnews.com/003069.html.

Reg's Natural You Tweaks

1. Let the Sun Shine In. Sensible exposure to natural sunlight, without putting any chemicals or chemically-stuffed sunscreen on at all, is the simplest and easiest—and one of the most important—strategies for improving your health. I urge you to read the book *The UV Advantage* by Dr. Michael Holick to get the full story on natural sunlight. You can find this book at most local and online bookstores. *Note: This is not a paid endorsement. I recommend it because of its of great importance in preventing chronic disease and enhancing health without drugs or surgery. If more people understood this information, we could drastically reduce the rates of chronic disease around the world.*

2. The Power of the Sun. Sunlight exposure is truly one of the most powerful healing therapies in the world. The healing power of natural sunlight is astonishing, and you can get it free of charge. That's why nobody's promoting it, of course.

- 32% of doctors and medical school students are vitamin D deficient
- 40% of the U.S. population is vitamin D deficient
- 42% of African American women of childbearing age are deficient in vitamin D
- 48% of young girls (9-11 years old) are vitamin D deficient
- Up to 60% of all hospital patients share vitamin D deficiency
- 76% of pregnant mothers are severely vitamin D deficient, causing widespread vitamin D deficiencies in their unborn children, which predisposes them to type 1 diabetes, arthritis, multiple sclerosis, and schizophrenia later in life. A whopping 81% of the children born to these mothers were vitamin D deficient.
- Up to 80% of nursing-home patients are vitamin D deficient.

Why does it matter if you are vitamin D deficient? Here is a list of diseases and conditions caused by vitamin D deficiency:

- Osteoporosis is commonly caused by a lack of vitamin D. Vitamin D deficiencies greatly impairs calcium absorption.[8]
- Sufficient vitamin D prevents prostate cancer, breast cancer, cancer, ovarian cancer, depression, and colon cancer.[9]
- "Rickets" is the name of a bone-wasting disease caused by vitamin D deficiency.
- Vitamin D deficiency may exacerbate type 2 diabetes and impair insulin production in the pancreas.[10]
- Obesity impairs vitamin D utilization in the body, meaning obese people need twice as much vitamin D.[11]
- Vitamin D is used around the world to treat psoriasis.[12]
- Vitamin D deficiency causes schizophrenia.[13]
- Seasonal Affective Disorder is caused by a melatonin imbalance initiated by lack of exposure to sunlight. Vitamin D supplementation has been shown to help alleviate the effects of Seasonal Affective Disorder.[14]
- Chronic vitamin D deficiency is often misdiagnosed as fibromyalgia because its symptoms are so similar: muscle weakness, aches, and pains.

---

[8] Holick, M. F. (2007). Vitamin D deficiency. *N Engl j Med*, 2007(357), 266-281.

[9] Garland, C. F., Garland, F. C., Gorham, E. D., Lipkin, M., Newmark, H., Mohr, S. B., & Holick, M. F. (2006). The role of vitamin D in cancer prevention. American journal of public health, 96(2), 252-261.

[10] Pittas, A. G., Lau, J., Hu, F. B., & Dawson-Hughes, B. (2007). The role of vitamin D and calcium in type 2 diabetes. A systematic review and meta-analysis. *The journal of clinical endocrinology & metabolism*, 92(6), 2017-2029.

[11] Wortsman, J., Matsuoka, L. Y., Chen, T. C., Lu, Z., & Holick, M. F. (2000). Decreased bioavailability of vitamin D in obesity. *The American journal of clinical nutrition*, 72(3), 690-693.

[12] Kragballe, K. (1992). Vitamin D analogues in the treatment of psoriasis. *Journal of cellular biochemistry*, 49(1), 46-52.

[13] McGrath, J., Saari, K., Hakko, H., Jokelainen, J., Jones, P., Järvelin, M. R., ... & Isohanni, M. (2004). Vitamin D supplementation during the first year of life and risk of schizophrenia: a Finnish birth cohort study. *Schizophrenia research*, 67(2), 237-245.

[14] Gloth 3rd, F. M., Alam, W., & Hollis, B. (1999). Vitamin D vs broad spectrum phototherapy in the treatment of seasonal affective disorder. *The journal of nutrition, health & aging*, 3(1), 5-7.

- Your risk of developing serious diseases like diabetes and cancer is reduced 50%–80% through simple, sensible exposure to natural sunlight 2-3 times each week.

I also want to share with you fifteen facts you probably never knew about vitamin D and sunlight exposure.[15] When you get out into the sun, you are exposing yourself to your external environment to create a healthier internal environment, and it's so simple. Here are some of the greatest benefits to letting the sun shine in:

1. As mentioned above, vitamin D prevents osteoporosis, depression, prostate cancer, breast cancer and even affects diabetes, and obesity. Vitamin D is perhaps the single most underrated nutrient in the world of nutrition. That's probably because it's free; your body makes it when sunlight touches your skin. Drug companies can't sell sunlight, so there's little promotion of its health benefits.

2. Vitamin D is produced by your skin in response to exposure to ultraviolet radiation from natural sunlight.

3. The healing rays of ordinary sunlight (that generate vitamin D in your skin) cannot penetrate glass. So, your body doesn't synthesize vitamin D when sitting in your car or home.

4. It is nearly impossible to get adequate amounts of vitamin D from your diet. Sunlight exposure is the only reliable way to generate vitamin D in your own body.

5. A person would have to drink ten tall glasses of vitamin D-fortified milk each day just to get minimum levels of vitamin D into their diet.

6. The further you live from the equator, the longer exposures you need for the sun to generate vitamin D. Canada, the UK, and most US states are far from the equator and therefore people living in these regions require longer periods of sun exposure.

---

[15] Holick, M. F. (2007). Vitamin D deficiency. *N Engl j Med*, 2007(357), 266-281.

7. People with dark skin pigmentation may need 20-30 times as much exposure to sunlight as fair-skinned people to generate the same amount of vitamin D. That's why prostate cancer is epidemic among black men—it's a simple, but widespread, sunlight deficiency.

8. Sufficient levels of vitamin D are crucial for calcium absorption in your intestines. Without enough vitamin D, your body cannot absorb calcium, rendering calcium supplements useless.

9. Chronic vitamin D deficiency cannot be reversed overnight; it takes months of vitamin D supplementation and sunlight exposure to rebuild the body's bones and nervous system.

10. Even weak sunscreens (SPF 8) block your body's ability to generate vitamin D by 95%. This is how sunscreen products cause disease—by creating a critical vitamin deficiency in the body. My advice is to avoid sunscreens altogether. Now I know making that statement causes endless uproar and discussion, but I stick to this advice, adhere to it myself, and ensure my clients do as well.

11. It is impossible to generate too much vitamin D in your body from sunlight exposure; your body will self-regulate and only generate what it needs.

12. If it hurts to press firmly on your sternum, you may be suffering from chronic vitamin D deficiency right now.

13. Vitamin D is "activated" in your body by your kidneys and liver before it can be used.

14. Having kidney disease or liver damage can greatly impair your body's ability to activate circulating vitamin D.

15. The sunscreen industry doesn't want you to know that your body needs sunlight exposure, because that realization would mean lower sales of sunscreen products.

Key Takeaways

Refined sugar is *not* food, and it's very dangerous to your body, your mind, and your life. Sugar substitutes are even more dangerous. Simple answer: use natural. It's safe, simple, and is perfect just the way it naturally comes!

Simply adding supplements like probiotics, enzymes, vitamin C, MSM, and vitamin D can rapidly improve your journey to becoming the best natural version of you.

One of the simplest things you can do to improve your health is to get outside and expose your bare skin to sunlight daily. Yes! I said it! Bare skin, real sun, nothing else. So, before you let your limiting beliefs and old ways of thinking take this amazing joy and powerful healing technique away from you, listen: vitamin D deficiencies cause many health problems, from depression to cancer. Chances are you are vitamin D deficient, so make sure you're spending enough time in the sun, especially if you live far from the equator, or if your skin is naturally dark.

If you haven't allowed your body to enjoy the sun for a while, then be smart and go slow. Start with just a couple of minutes a few times a day, then slowly increase your time in the sun. Your body loves it, wants it, and needs it, so once you get used to being in the sun, the fears, worries and issues will go away. Remember, be smart! You're going to expose your natural body to natural elements, so make sure the natural stuff you're putting in and on your body all work in harmony. Don't fill your body with a bunch of chemically-based, processed stuff, then lather chemically-based, processed stuff on your skin when spending time in the sun. Common sense, education, and awareness all create harmony, health, and happiness.

"

There is more wisdom in
your body than in your
deepest philosophies.

—FRIEDRICH NIETZCHE

Body Wisdom

Did you know that if you just put you first, you can make more money, be happier, healthier, be more successful, be more fulfilled, get more done, and have more free time? If I've piqued your interest, keep reading to find out how and why.

What does your body need, and what are the best practices that enhance, empower, repair, restore, and rejuvenate? I work with individuals to do all this from the inside and out. We work together analyzing and monitoring their bodies, their environments, and their relationships to look for strengths, imbalances, weaknesses, or injuries so they can develop a plan of action that best supports them in their ultimate physical and mental performance, needs, and goals. Throughout this book, my goal has been to do the same with you.

You may wonder why I mentioned mental performance when speaking about the body's needs. When your body is given the proper nourishment, rest, strengthening, and attention, then it responds and communicates to your brain and different interconnected systems in a very efficient and powerful way.

Take, for example, someone who has digestive issues often (indigestion, heart burn, diarrhea, constipation, cramps, pain, weight gain, weight loss and such) and does a little research, asks all their friends, goes to see a few doctors, and "specialists." Someone in the media could simply point out that they don't have the proper gut flora in their intestines, and you can witness millions and millions of people rushing out to buy this stuff to fix their issue. But, it could also mean they are eating too much processed food and not enough fresh foods. Maybe they are not getting enough sleep and their body is just too exhausted to actually do the job it needs to do. They may have a toxic overload. They might possibly be taking medications or other supplements that don't live in harmony together. Or, their stomach problems could be due to stress, the wrong type of exercising, toxic overload, bad food combinations, too much or too little of something, bad relationships or bad environments, or other causes.

When unaddressed, root causes like I listed above can lead to stomach pain, back pain, leg aches, headaches, concentration difficulties, mood swings, memory troubles, weight gain, low energy, skin issues, lack of hunger, brain fog, and/or overwhelm from everyday life. A simpler solution to all of those symptoms could be to take a step back to clearly see all aspects of your life and how everything affects everything else. This is also why getting your personal health advice from a Facebook buddy or out of some health or fitness magazine is downright wrong for you. Changing your diet by adding in cultured foods, which help grow healthy gut flora,[1] may be the right way to deal with this issue for some, but becoming aware of how everything affects everything and clearly listening to your own body, your intuition, your emotions, and your common sense will guide you to exactly the right choices for you.

What is Body Wisdom?

Body Wisdom is a relationship between the body, mind, beliefs, and environment. The body is our tool to experience the world. What a lot of people may not know is that we can use the messages our body sends us to guide us in making the best choices that will result in the best versions of ourselves.

Our culture today has created a hive mind, so to speak—if something isn't working in the body, then we focus on the specific body part to fix, or find a pill or potion to take. How I approach my work with people is the complete opposite. I use the body's messages as an indicator and guide people to look at the whole system (the person's beliefs, choices, and

---

[1] *Why Fermented Foods May Be the Next Big Antidepressant.* (2015, November 6) All Body Ecology Articles. Retrieved August 07, 2017 from https://bodyecology.com/articles/fermented-foods-antidepressant.

lifestyle). The journey to becoming the best version of you then becomes a map of your life. That map begins with the body, and its compass, Body Wisdom, will give you the mission and directions you need to follow in order to achieve a life that is fulfilling, successful, and healthy.

Heal Your Body

Your body may need healing, even if you don't have any physical injuries or issues that you are yet aware of. You know your body has healing capabilities, but you may not quite have realized the power behind that wisdom.

> Take time for yourself each day and maintain the wellbeing of your body and mind the same way you do with your clothes, house, or car.

Often, I hear people telling me, "I'm in perfect health, I don't need to think about healing or repairing my body." This is like saying, "I already know everything and there is no point in educating myself anymore." Or, "I just tuned up my car and put new oil and filters in it, now all I have to do is drive it for the rest of my life." Thinking you can just keep 'driving' your body without consistently doing maintenance to keep your high levels of mental and physical performance is simply empowering ailment and illness to grow. If you are not consistently supporting and helping to heal your body, then you are going backwards. Every day you are getting older, putting your body under stress and pressure, and making your body do more work. Every day you need to work with your body and support it if you're going to live a long and healthy life, and if you want to continue consistently doing the things you love to do. You may already be sick or injured without knowing it. Learning to build a body that is capable of healing itself does not require prescription medicine, but it is a daily requirement.

The Natural You approach provides the steps to support natural healing in the body. Recognizing the *need* to heal continually and consistently (without prescription medicine) is the first important step to doing something about it. For your body to heal every day, this approach requires you to build a new relationship with your body and your awareness of its daily needs.

Learn to become in tune with your body, and don't put the little things off, because they have a nasty habit of turning into big things quite quickly. What do I mean by that? I mean that you can stop having to "deal with it"! Many of my clients turn to me when things get so bad that they "can't deal with it anymore." That is my point exactly! Why wait? You would be better off if you stopped learning to "deal with" the small things, the little messages that your body and mind tell you regularly.

Take time for yourself each day and maintain the wellbeing of your body and mind the same way you do with your clothes, house, or car. Just like you perform regular maintenance on your car or HVAC or the exterior of your house, you need to be maintaining yourself. If you do this, you'll minimize the chances of having to "deal with" more severe issues later.

Even then, at some point, your body will inevitably need healing and repair. Human beings cannot avoid this. At some point, you will strain or injure yourself while exercising or moving, or you will need help recovering from an illness or medical condition. It will be much easier to heal and repair if you've already been taking care of your body daily. You hear this all the time from doctors of fit and healthy patients who experience traumatic injuries. Those patients heal quickly because they've been taking care of their bodies. Don't wait—take the little steps today that will make a big difference in the long term.

Are You in Need of Healing Now?

Let me ask you this: do you ever feel great?

Do you ever feel full of energy, on top of the world, powerful, and confident?

Are you ever able to wake up naturally in the morning, without an alarm clock and jump out of bed with a spring in your step, ready to take on your day, no matter what comes your way?

Are you able to go through your entire day without any aches, pains, cramps, concentration problems, negative stress, energy loss, or mood swings?

If you answered yes to every question, great! You are experiencing exceptionally high levels of health and wellbeing. But, are you able to feel like this every day? If you don't feel strong and full of energy almost every day, then your body needs healing, even if you don't have any physical injuries or ailments that you are aware of.

Here are a few more questions you should ask yourself to assess your health:

- Do you have aches and pains (even minor ones), allergies, skin irritations or spots, ringing in the ears, or spots in front of your eyes?

- Do you sleep poorly, or sleep deeply but wake up tired? Do you feel tired all day, even if you slept all night *and* had an afternoon nap?

- Do you have frequent and/or large mood swings? Do you feel like a grouchy grizzly bear but don't really know why?

- Do you sometimes struggle to think clearly or concentrate properly?

- Is your memory not as good as it used to be?

If you answered yes to any of these questions, it's an indicator that your body is toxic, your muscles aren't working as well as they could and should, and most or all your body's systems are "out of order."

Healing the Natural Way

Healing the "natural way" is about becoming aware of how everything affects everything, and your choice and power to control it. Educating yourself and incorporating vital yet subtle key changes to your routine will create massive improvements to your life, health, and performance levels. Detoxing, improving your external and internal environments, learning how your beliefs contribute to how well you care for yourself and how much success you enjoy, and taking responsibility to get to know your body and its messages will support you in achieving and maintaining all you have been looking for.

How can you learn to naturally enjoy the following?

- High levels of natural energy

Reg's Natural You Tweaks

1. Massage. Our bodies are nourished by touch, so getting a really great massage by a highly-qualified and naturally-talented therapist, at least once or twice a month, can be a great addition to your *Natural You* routine. A knowledgeable and aware therapist, trained in many different modalities, with the ability to 'feel' what's going on through the various systems living in your body, can enhance all aspects of your body and mind. Expert touch in certain places on your body causes biochemical changes, and those changes bring on healing and release negativity.

There is plenty of scientific research to support the idea that proper massage stimulates the body's parasympathetic nervous system,[1] which reduces the risk of or the effects of high blood pressure[2]—a rampant illness in our society. Deep-tissue massage helps your muscles remain supple yet strong and prevents injury and strain due to too much muscular tension. Massage can even be self-administered, and research shows that even if you're no 'expert,' you can still get to know your own body and enjoy the great benefits from just instinctively applying mild pressure and massaging yourself. Try it out with your fingertips, hands, arms, and feet near the areas that are hurting or just need some love, and in certain key places like the sides of your neck, your head, along your eyebrows, your ears, biceps, and triceps, and your hands, legs, and feet. You can experience for yourself how gentle rubbing and digging around can help you to understand what's going on in your body, and make it feel great too.

2. Muscle Balancing. Muscle balancing targets imbalances in your body due to strong muscles pulling on weak or injured ones, which is both a symptom and a cause of less-than-optimal health.

---

[1] Diego, M. A., & Field, T. (2009). Moderate pressure massage elicits a parasympathetic nervous system response. *International Journal of Neuroscience*, 119(5), 630-638.

[2] Aourell, M., Skoog, M., & Carleson, J. (2005). Effects of Swedish massage on blood pressure. *Complementary therapies in clinical practice*, 11(4), 242-246.

Invasive medical procedures and pharmaceuticals are not needed for muscle balancing therapy; in fact, they often make it worse. You should consult a respected source to analyze your body, work the imbalances, and provide a proper training program to correct the issues long before allowing anyone to start cutting you.

I can't tell you how many thousands of people I have met that have either received an un-needed operation for something that could have been easily rebalanced by the right therapist. Those people are now living in damaged bodes and are in pain for the rest of their lives. Alternatively, I have witnessed countless individuals who try a different, alternative option while waiting for an operation and were "miraculously cured," no operation needed. Educate yourself and truly get to the core of your issues before allowing anyone to cut or destroy anything in your body.

3. Body Alignment. This is a gentle therapeutic practice which may involve osteopath-type therapy. It can help relieve many aches and pains, including sciatic pain and headaches, and is known to help enhance energy flow throughout the body.

4. Organ Balancing. This is a holistic approach to healing aches, pains, and nervous system-related conditions in the body. A vast array of painful and debilitating conditions may be treatable with organ balancing. When done correctly, it is one of the most powerful and enlightening therapies you will ever experience.

Please note that you should always consult experts in the field and licensed practitioners before you sign on for any listed body-healing remedy. Check out your practitioner carefully before committing.

- Enhanced performance

- Your perfect weight

- Ultimate health (free from chronic ailments, pains, and disease)

- A fast and powerful mind

- Active aging (the ability to dance, travel, make love, and enjoy life—long beyond your golden years)

- A great business life

- An amazing family life

- Time to do what you want

We've already covered some of the foundations for healthier living, including beliefs and environment. Now, it's time to look at how to sustain the lifestyle that's right for you.

Another approach to healing your body naturally is through physical movement. Moving your body will improve mood, flexibility, vitality, and strength. It's why doctors and therapists want you to get up and move around very soon after a hip replacement, birth, or cast removal. Movement uses your body's wisdom to learn what kind of movement works best for your mind and body as a whole.

Work Your Body

To get and stay healthy, you need the right type of exercise or movement in the right way. Exercise means different things to different people. We all have different ways we enjoy working out and keeping fit, whether it is working out hard in a gym or at home, or whether we prefer to find alternative methods of toning our bodies and keeping our muscles healthy and balanced.

The 10 Keys to Ultimate Health, Happiness, and Success are designed to work with each other. It's a systematic approach to life and it's completely individualized, unlike other programs you've tried.

The fitness and movement programs I provide my clients are custom-designed to fit their personality type, body, lifestyle, needs, and goals.

Ultimately, when devising an exercise plan, you should look at the following factors:

- Your beliefs around what exercise means to you, and why you do it

- Your body and its current physical capabilities, as well as the goals you have for top physical performance

- The foods and liquids you are choosing that support or inhibit your fitness goals

- Your awareness of whether your body needs detoxification to improve your fitness results

- What exercises you enjoy, and when you enjoy doing them

After looking at the relationship a person has with movement, fitness, and exercise, I design a plan that can be done anytime, anywhere. My goal is to set you up for success to maintain the level of movement your body needs at work, at home and while traveling. When the body feels taken care of (what I call Body Wisdom), it will create chemicals that will produce feelings of power, peace, relaxation, confidence, and happiness. Your thoughts will become more positive, and it will become easy to maintain a lifestyle that makes you feel great.

Do you see how everything works together?

"But I can't do it!" "My doctor said I shouldn't." "It hurts when I do it . . ." There are endless excuses, and they are just that—uneducated limiting beliefs and fears. If you have injuries, chronic pain, or physical issues, it's important to spend some time educating yourself about the best types of movement for your body, in the ways that your body CAN do it. The key is to move your body, not lay on the couch or sit in a chair for long periods of time. You must find the way to support and train your body and mind so it can perform in the most efficient, nourishing ways. Working your body doesn't have to feel stressful or dull. It doesn't need to be aggressive, painful, or monotonous. It's fun to have fun, so enjoy whatever it is you are doing to make your body look and feel great. Just have fun, be creative, and enjoy variety—especially when you move.

Most of us know that we should work our bodies. It makes us feel more alive, more energized, less stressed, and sexier. You know that physical activity is important to your health. But, a great many of you just aren't working your bodies like you could or should. It seems to become harder to do as we get older—but even a great many teenagers and college undergraduates don't seem to manage it very well. Why are so many, as a society, not doing what we should with exercise, especially since it is supposed to bring all these good things to our lives?

One of the main reasons why people don't get moving often enough is that their beliefs and the drivers behind their choices are messed up. Another reason is that they may be doing an activity that doesn't fit their lifestyle, or that they just don't enjoy. Many people do the wrong type of exercise for the wrong reason, and at the wrong time for their body type. Then, they do the exercises the wrong way, causing all sorts of other problems and issues.

For example, let's say that starting today, I insist you start doing yoga! You will be adding yoga to your schedule every day for the next year. Where did your beliefs take you? When I said "yoga," did you get excited about trying something new, or did you instantly shut me out and come up with 10 reasons why you "can't" or "won't"?

"It's too difficult to fit studio classes into my busy life," you say. A better alternative would be to set up a quick, at-home and in-office workout that leaves you feeling great when you're done. You can do this in seven to 10 minutes flat.

"But," you say, "I can't do yoga. It's against my religion. It's too hard. I can't touch my toes, stand on my head, or scratch my bum with my nose. So, there is no point even starting to try, right?"

Wrong!

Yoga is all about you and your relationship with your body. When you start slow, you start to feel your body, reintroduce your brain to your body, and allow them to get to know each-other again. You will be amazed at what your body can actually do, and you will be very happy with how quickly your body changes, and how fast aches, pains and issues 'magically' disappear. You can exercise your entire body, with no equipment at all, anytime, anywhere, for free!

Given the importance of staying active, doesn't it make sense that you need to choose an activity that you can learn to do properly, so that you can enjoy it and can stick with consistently, no matter where you are, and regardless of your time limitations?

I work with the busiest people on this planet, from world leaders to small family leaders. We are all busy. Yet, when we're guided in the right way, we all have the time to do all the things we should do, while doing all the things we have to, while enjoying all the things we can and want to do. It all comes down to beliefs and choices. The great thing about beliefs and choices is that they can always change.

Forget the Fitness Goals!

If your fitness regimen is going to support you in achieving the body, energy levels, confidence, and great health you want long term, then forget the goals! We constantly hear about the new goals people set. These goals might include losing 10 pounds this month, becoming stronger and putting on some more muscle, looking better in your clothes or on the beach, becoming more energized, increasing the distance you are able to hike, swim, or walk at one time, improving your bicycling speed by the end of the month, or anything related to your personal health, fitness, and wellness. Those all sound great, but a goal is something you may or may not achieve, may or may not remember, and may or may not give any importance to. Most likely, your goals, like your New Year's resolutions, often cause more stress and frustration then not having them at all. I say become aware. When you put yourself first, focus on the tiny, easy-to-implement and consistent changes and choices, you will achieve results way beyond any goals you set.

Do you think that your performance at work would improve if you had more energy, felt better, and could think more clearly with better memory?

Do you believe that if you felt better more often, you could skip all those appointments with doctors and "specialists," get off the medications, have more energy, do the things you love to do, have more passion, and do everything you do to the best of your ability? Do you think it would make a difference in the way people perceive and value you? Do you think it would help people have more respect for you and treat you better? Do you think you would enjoy spending time around people more, and they would enjoy being around you more?

The answer is yes—and that would ultimately lead to more opportunities, more enjoyment in what you do, and it would help you earn more money, allowing you to do more of the things you really want to do.

Is it worth the effort?

You had better believe it. Yes, it is! But, that is just my opinion. What do you believe?

All your fitness and life choices need to be SMART: Specific, Measurable, Attainable, Realistic and True to You. SMART is an acronym that you can use to guide your choices. Every minute of every day you are making choices that either take you toward or away from where you want to be and what you want to achieve. It's the little consistent choices that make the biggest differences. SMART choices are your key to achieving and maintaining great health, happiness, success, and high levels of mental and physical performance. Using SMART choices can be the key to effectively living a life that empowers you, helping you achieve your 'wants' and 'needs' faster, and maintaining them longer.

There is no need to spend an hour or three in the gym every day. You can be fit and healthy just by being active and doing things around your home, office, hotel room, on the local street, or in the park, saving you more time and money, by simply finding ways to fit more movement into your everyday life.

If you are a pro athlete, or you want to be, by all means, spend the hours at the gym needed to meet your goals. That is a totally different

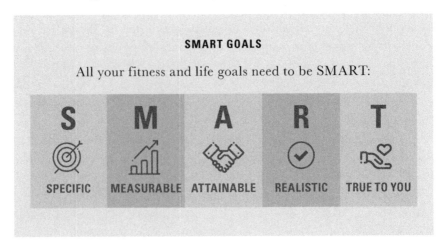

SMART GOALS

All your fitness and life goals need to be SMART:

S	M	A	R	T
SPECIFIC	MEASURABLE	ATTAINABLE	REALISTIC	TRUE TO YOU

lifestyle, where your main focus all day, every day is to achieve that exceptionally high level of performance. But, if you wish to achieve greatness and maintain it long term, and you are dedicated to being the best at whatever it is you are doing, you must include all the other areas of your entire life. Balance is power, and imbalance managed in the right way can secure long term balance. If you focus on one goal while ignoring all the other vital keys in your life, you could be leaving the best of who you are on the bench.

Make choices that are specifically for you, that fit into your lifestyle and schedule, and that are enjoyable to you. Then, stay alert and pay attention to how everything affects everything. When you start living smart, things become easy and all the effort you put in will give you much better results. Whatever plans you make to build and maintain your fitness, make sure they're SMART.

Another thing to keep in mind is the people who will be supporting you to keep consistently making SMART choices. Consider hiring a properly-trained and professional coach, mentor, therapist, nutritionist, and/or personal trainer with the right knowledge, experience, talent, and passion for what they are doing. Get to know them, interview their clients, and watch how they work with others. Having the right support will minimize the risk of injury or burnout and save you from any beliefs that are working against you, bad lifestyle choices, unhealthy environments, improper exercising, muscle imbalance, and improper fuel intake. You need to be the expert when it comes to your body. Then, when you work with other experts, you will be very clear about what your body wants and needs. By having the right support, you will ensure you are doing all you must do in order to effectively and efficiently achieve your wants and needs and maintain them long term.

Plus, when you're paying the 'right' someone to keep you on track, you will have someone who is 100% there for you and your best interests, not for their bank account. The right professional will want you to succeed as much or more then you do. They will encourage you, empower you, and sometimes kick your butt, and you'll be more motivated to work toward your wants and needs. Avoid "specialists," coaches, mentors, therapists, and personal trainers who have taken some weekend courses, are in training and are not looking, living and achieving the way you want. These are not professionals to trust your body, life and future with.

Reg's Natural You Tweaks

1. Get the Right Help. The most important thing before starting any health or fitness program is to be clear on what you really want, and why you want it. So many people pump money into a local gym, health food store, fad diet, or home gym equipment. They start programs without clear intentions. This usually leads to them quitting in frustration after failing to lose weight or other benchmarks.

Before you start, get together with a life coach, a personal fitness trainer, a sports therapist, and/or a nutrition expert—someone who has the knowledge to help you formulate SMART choices. You are the one who knows your body, your lifestyle, and your needs. Be bold and tell your trainer or coach what you like to do best, and make sure they include those exercises in your plan. Telling your coach what you enjoy can also help to motivate your coach and support you both to hold you accountable for getting the results you want. If you don't want to go to a gym, don't. Be SMART! There are endless ways to be fit and healthy without ever stepping foot in a gym.

Remember, a great coach will understand your body, your personality type, your lifestyle, and how you can achieve what you really want and need. They'll watch and monitor exactly how your body is moving and functioning, and they'll watch your training techniques and timing. If there are injuries, imbalances, or energy issues, they will guide you to repair and rebalance rather than sending you away or telling you to push through it. The right mentor and coach will know when and how to push you, while maintaining the protection you need so as to not push to far. The intention is to cross goal lines, break barriers, question beliefs, make smart choices, and do everything possible to ensure you achieve exactly what you want, and show you the balanced and efficient way to get more while maintaining everything you have.

2. Interview Your Trainer or Coach. Just because they have a certificate hanging on the wall doesn't mean they know what they are doing. And, if they are highly skilled at what they do, they may not really know how to teach you to do it, but in the way your body needs it. In fact, from my experience around the world, it is very rare to find a great coach or trainer, so take your time. Check them out thoroughly. Watch them work with other clients and interview their clients. What do their clients look like? Are they healthy, fit, and pain-free? Have their clients regularly hit their weekly, monthly, and yearly goals working with this "specialist" or "professional"? Does this person who is going to help you look and feel great actually look and feel great themselves? When the trainer is working with their clients, are they 100% focused on the clients, or are they chatting with others, playing on their phone, or lost in some sort of daydream? Get very clear on exactly what you want and why, then surround yourself with the right people to get you there.

Enjoy It and Have Fun!

I can't emphasize this enough: it's essential to enjoy your life, even in the serious cases and situations. When you have fun and you enjoy what you're doing, or at least put your best positive energy, passion, and intention into whatever it is you do, your entire experience changes. Many people don't work out because they find it to be dull and boring. Others claim they don't have time or believe they just can't do it, or they think exercise isn't very important. They don't like the same old routine week in, week out, or they don't like the environment they go train in, so they lose their mental focus. Who can stay mentally focused at that intensity doing anything if they are bored, not wanting to be where they are, or don't believe it is really worth their time and effort? Without a strong mental focus, clarity, and passion, driven by your desire to achieve the best possible outcome, it's very difficult to stay sufficiently motivated to do anything really well, or to the best of your ability.

> Without a strong mental focus, clarity, and passion, driven by your desire to achieve the best possible outcome, it's very difficult to stay sufficiently motivated to do anything really well, or to the best of your ability.

Many people fail to achieve their goals, or work out and stay active and fit as they should, because they simply aren't clear on their why's, how's and when's. What kind of physical activities do they really enjoy doing, or could they learn to enjoy if they just found the right way for them to do it? If the thought of doing one more push-up fills you with dread, soon you will find that you quit your exercise regimen again—and your health will suffer for it.

Most people start fitness programs and quit after a short time. Why? Because they are doing something they don't enjoy, and they're probably doing it in the wrong way for them. People are running when they really want to be walking or swimming when they really want to be dancing. Some don't do anything because any kind of strenuous physical activity makes them give up before they start. So many times, I hear people say,

"I can't do that." What a terrible belief! They have failed before even trying to start. So many go through their entire life like this, avoiding and creating fear around anything and everything outside of their immediate comfort zone.

> Many people fail to achieve their goals, or work out and stay active and fit as they should, because they simply aren't clear on their why's, how's and when's.

Let's think about yoga again as an example. I know I used this example earlier, but for me it is a constant when talking about health, wellness, physical and mental enhancement. I'm consistently telling people who want to eliminate chronic aches and pains, mental pressures and frustration, while at the same time reconnecting with their bodies and learning to appreciate them, to do yoga. But, 99.99% of the time, I get negativity rather than optimistic hope, with the excitement to learn something new.

Why do you believe that is? Why are people generally so negative about anything they don't fully understand, know what is really involved, or know how to make it their own? So many times, we categorize things just because of what we have heard, or learned from others. Yoga doesn't mean you go to your first class and do a head stand or a back flip. Yoga is all about you, your body, and starting from where you are. If you can breathe and move your body, you can do yoga! You start right where you are, how you are, and every day you do a little more. Before you know it, you are easily doing the things you initially thought you couldn't!

It's so important to discover how to move and use your body, then learn to move and use it right, and then do it consistently, here and now. Start where you are, then improve little by little from there. Every day you will feel better and you'll be able to do better. There's no pressure, no forcing it, no competition or judgment, no points to keep, no one to impress and no group effort required. Just enjoy the process and the excitement from noticing your own improvements and growth—it's that simple. And, the great thing is that there are no limits. You don't have to do just one thing or one type of exercise. Get adventurous, have fun, and enjoy yourself. This is all about you, your time, and your life. LOVE IT!

Who said that exercise has to be painful, difficult, hard work, boring, or the same old dull routine? You're human and you need fun, creativity, and variety—*especially* when working out. Besides, once your body's musculoskeletal system gets too used to a routine, your real advances diminish. Your body needs variety in its exercise activities to get optimal results, to help you keep getting stronger and to consistently improve your body, or, at the very least, maintain what you have so you don't consistently find yourself in an older, weaker, sicker body that makes it very difficult to enjoy life in, and do all the things you want and need to do.

> ## Instead, I teach many ways to build a strong, healthy, fit body using little or no fitness equipment, little or no money and very little time, and that can be incorporated into anyone's daily routine and hectic lifestyle.

Don't buy into your own lies and excuses! Stop believing that you can't get motivated and moving because you don't have access to a gym, or believing any other excuse. That is absolutely untrue and a complete fabrication to support you in your own failures! You can get the same benefits from creating a routine at home as you would get at the gym. In fact, 80% or more of my clients do not enjoy working out in the gym, and never step foot into one. Instead, I teach many ways to build a strong, healthy, fit body using little or no fitness equipment, little or no money and very little time, and that can be incorporated into anyone's daily routine and hectic lifestyle.

A fun workout regimen for any individual is largely subjective, not one-size-fits-all. But here are a few ideas to help you get moving that have been popular with my clients:

- Get involved in a local or international training group or club—a great way to see new places, meet new people and have fun!

- Start your own club or group. It's easy to find others who want to feel great too.

- Plant a garden. Digging in the dirt and pulling weeds are great exercise and clear your mind!

- Hike a mountain or try trail hiking.

- Go mountain biking.

- Train for and do bicycle spring racing.

- Play racquetball.

- Play volleyball.

- Go rowing and kayaking if you live near water.

- Exercise with a medicine ball.

- Try Zumba dancing. I bet you can't do a class without laughing uncontrollably.

- Do martial arts self-defense training and conditioning. Mixed martial arts is a lot of fun and a great way to blow off some steam!

- Go swimming.

- Get involved in adventure travel and sports. It's a great way to discover new towns, new neighborhoods, or new countries.

- Check out your local park. Is there some kind of class going on?

- Go power walking.

- Be adventurous. See how many ways you can reach the same destination without going the same way twice.

- Use bungee cords to exercise anywhere.

- Build something.

- Go help others do things, with no expectations in return. It is very empowering.

The above list just contains a handful of basic ideas to spark your own, and you may well have some different ones. What's important is that you keep your physical activity regimen fun and filled with mental interest and variety so that you do it consistently. Couple that with SMART choices and guidance, and you cannot fail to feel your body getting healthier and stronger while you start living your dreams. Your body and mind are directly connected and will be naturally inspired through physical movement, enhancing and empowering every aspect of your life. So, get up, get out and get moving now.

Cancer Care and Prevention

Mounting research shows the benefits of physical movement for people diagnosed with cancer, depression, chronic aches and pains, fatigue, and so much more, including reductions in recurrence of chronic ailments and mortality.[2] Exercise 'prescriptions' are an essential part of cancer care! I consistently get my clients to spend as much time as possibly they can near water and nature, walking barefoot as much as possible and absorb Mother Nature's natural medicine. The clients that do this immediately feel and experience dramatic and positive developments.

What do you think?

Millions of cancer patients can reap the powerful and natural benefits from SMART choices, lifestyle changes, and physical exercise, and they can do so safely.[3] Physical exercise helps you gain strength, tone your body, get your blood flowing, oxygenate your body and mind with clean, fresh, natural air, and support your immune system by helping it to flush out the toxins, which in turn empowers it to clean out more and clear your mind and empower your thoughts. This is especially important when so many people—including many cancer patients— are depressed, scared, confused, frustrated, overweight, or obese. All of these different negative elements are risk factors for cancer, making

---

[2] Galvão, D. A., & Newton, R. U. (2005). Review of exercise intervention studies in cancer patients. Journal of clinical oncology, 23(4), 899-909.

[3] Harpham, W. (2010). *Delivering Patient-Centered Care to Cancer Survivors: The Critical Role of Communication.* 5th Biennial Cancer Survivorship Research Conference.

exercise even more important in cancer prevention. According to Julia Rowland, Ph.D., Director of the National Cancer Institute's Office of Cancer Survivorship, the new emphasis on exercise and weight control for cancer patients is the result of a mushrooming body of research aimed at helping cancer survivors live healthier lives.

In the Netherlands, cancer patients have access to specialized exercise programs. These programs exist because exercise is very beneficial for most patients before, during, and after treatment. Most health care insurers pay for the costs. Even some large companies pay for these programs since cancer patients feel better and go back to work faster when they have followed this exercise program. Dutch research is in progress to "prove" the added value of specialized exercise programs to cancer care, with variations in the intensity of the exercises and in-patient groups (regarding form of treatment). So yes, exercise prescriptions should definitely be part of cancer reversal.

> If the best scientists in the world are prescribing exercise to help prevent cancer, and as part of a cancer treatment plan, shouldn't you do it?

I absolutely believe that an exercise 'prescription,' combined with energy and physical balancing bodywork, clean nutrition, detoxification, SMART lifestyle changes, environmental education, and beliefs reassessment should be part of every treatment and recovery plan for those who have already been diagnosed with cancer—*and* for all those who do not ever want to go through having it. There are incredible gains to be had from breathing exercises like Pranayama and Laughter Yoga that would not put a fragile physiology at risk of injury or damage of any kind. Just like I've taught throughout the book, there is a way to create an individualized plan for any person based on their unique needs, even when those needs are greatly impacted by ailment or disability.

According to Dr. Otto Warburg, President of the Institute of Cell Physiology and Nobel Prize Winner, "Exercise and deep breathing techniques increase oxygen to the cells and are the most important factors in living a disease-free and energetic life. When cells get enough oxygen, cancer will not and cannot occur."[4] (Dr. Warburg is the only person ever to win the Nobel Prize for Medicine twice, and he was nominated for a third.) If the best scientists in the world are prescribing exercise to help prevent cancer, and as part of a cancer treatment plan, shouldn't you do it?

> Reconnect with your body and reconnect with yourself. You will love how discovering the real you will empower and enhance every aspect of who you are and how you live.

Your Body Knows Best

Healing the body doesn't have to be complicated. Learning what messages your body expresses to you through pain, dis-ease, and lack of mobility gives you an opportunity to discover an enjoyable way to nourish your body's needs. Physical movement you love to do is key to restore, rejuvenate, and regain the energy, strength, and natural healing qualities your body offers you. Your body is wiser than you think; all you need to do is listen. Reconnect with your body and reconnect with yourself. You will love how discovering the real you will empower and enhance every aspect of who you are and how you live.

---

[4] Gendry, S. *8 Scientists' Quotes on Laughter and Breathing.* Retrieved from http://www.laughteronlineuniversity.com/8-scientists-quotes-laughter-breathing/.

Key Takeaways

When your body is given the right energy, environment, proper nourishment, excitement, rest, strengthening, and attention, it responds to and communicates with your brain and different interconnected systems in a very powerful and efficient way.

Learn to take time for yourself each day and maintain the wellbeing of your body and mind the same way you do with your pets, house, or car.

Healing the "natural way" is about making subtle, easy key changes to your routine to create massive improvements to your life, health, and performance levels.

Physically moving your body will improve your health, energy, mood, flexibility, vitality, and strength.

Find a fitness and exercise routine that you *enjoy* and learn to enjoy adventure, near or far, energetic or relaxing. Adventuring will keep your mind healthy, relaxed, clear, and empowered, and it will keep your body active and healthy. You'll be more likely to stick with it if you do things that excite and inspire you. Take the time to consider what activities you actually take pleasure in doing, and do more of those things. Open up your imagination to doing things you never thought you could or would, or get going at something you have always wanted to do but have consistently put it off.

Use SMART choices and qualified professionals to help motivate, guide, and support you to reach the fitness and life level you desire.

When the body feels taken care of (Body Wisdom), it will create chemicals that will produce feelings of peace, relaxation, and happiness, and your thoughts, energy, and results will become more positive and powerful. Body Wisdom makes it easy to maintain a lifestyle that makes you feel great.

"

Tell me what you
eat, and I will tell you
what you are.

—G.K. CHESTERTON

Fuel Your Body with What It Needs

It's no secret that eating well will support your overall health. When I talk about nutrition, I always emphasize the relationship you have with the food you are choosing to fuel your body with. When looking at nutrition and your relationship with food, you must remember that there are no such things as "right" or "wrong" foods. There are foods that support the best version of you, and there are foods that will take away from that. Different foods have different effects on different people for different reasons, meaning everyone has a different relationship with food, and no one diet will ever work for everyone.[1]

Eating is one source of great health and high energy on the one hand, and great illness, fatigue, and an early grave on the other. It all depends on what and when you choose to eat and drink, and what products you choose to use in your home, and for what reasons. Unfortunately, the misinformation out there has expanded into such a vast sea that making the right choices (which used to be instinctive to even the most average human being) has become a daunting task for the majority. But, it doesn't need to be this way.

The terrible irony is that today, there are "health foods" being marketed to people which really aren't healthy foods at all. Many "health products" today are even worse than the supposedly unhealthy

---

[1] Sample, I. (2016, June 10). *Bespoke diets based on gut microbes could help beat disease and obesity.* Retrieved from https://www.theguardian.com/science/2015/jun/10/personalised-diets-diabetes-obesity-heart-disease-microbes-microbiomes.

foods that they are intended to replace. If you have ever tried to diet and started eating and drinking these "health foods" and found yourself failing, frustrated and disgusted, you can now start to understand why.

> Remember from earlier chapters that one of the most important factors when you're working to be healthier is finding changes that are *sustainable for your lifestyle*, enjoyable, and maintainable.

Developing a healthy and educated relationship with food is what optimal nutrition is about. There is a massive difference between filling and fueling your body, which absolutely affects every aspect of your life, health, happiness, and success. Clients who work with me specifically on nutrition find a balance between eating the foods they love and eating the foods that optimize overall performance. Remember from earlier chapters that one of the most important factors when you're working to be healthier is finding changes that are *sustainable for your lifestyle*, enjoyable, and maintainable. If you could never in a million years stick with a vegan diet, I'm not going to tell you that you should follow one.

Everyone's nutritional needs are unique and there is no reason you need to feel you must follow the same nutrition program as everyone else because it's the latest fad or because the world is pressuring you to do so. In fact, I work with my clients to design a program that is completely individualized and customized to meet their specific needs, for their lifestyle and their body. My nutrition programs have supported people in repairing and restoring leptin levels and blood sugar levels, eliminating toxins, empowering their minds, and reversing illness. Those programs have also helped people to work towards avoiding and eliminating allergies, ailments, and illnesses completely. When you avoid the one-size-fits-all approaches that you see featured all the time in the media and instead follow an approach that's best for *you*, you'll see amazing results, too, without the costs, frustration, and stress.

So how do you create an optimized, individualized life-enhancing plan for you? To start, you must learn to empower, restore, and cultivate the complex relationship you have with food and yourself. When I work with a client, we begin by looking at how their relationship with food impacts other areas of their life, and how other areas of their life impact the foods they crave or choose to eat. We explore how beliefs, environment, relationships, career, and Body Wisdom can contribute to the food choices they make.

The 10 Keys to Ultimate Happiness, Success, and Health all work together—the magic is in the awareness and actions you can begin taking while becoming the best version of you. It's the small steps that make the biggest long-term impact. You don't always need to see the destination, and often times what you believe you want to achieve changes while you're on the journey. So, relax and enjoy the process. Choose to be more aware, choose to start educating yourself, choose to make consistent choices daily that bring you closer to the lifestyle you wish to live, and choose to love who you are now, while being grateful for where you are so that you know where you need to move from. Before you know it, you will be well beyond what you ever believed could be possible.

> My nutrition programs have supported people in repairing and restoring leptin levels and blood sugar levels, eliminating toxins, empowering their minds, and reversing illness.

How Are You Fueling Your Body?

You cannot ignore the impact of change. Your body demands and needs certain types of food and drink—there's just no way around it. When approaching your relationship with food, it's important to focus on being happy and having a healthy, clean diet that empowers you. Choose foods and ways of cooking that ignite your passion and make you jump out of bed with excitement in the morning. Whatever your goals—weight loss, increased energy, drastic changes, achieving high levels and results, or overall improved body and health image to enhance your brand value— you have the power to create a healthy lifestyle that allows you to be the best version of you, in ways that are far more simple, empowering, and enhancing than you have been led to believe. What you choose to fuel your body with directly and impressively affects everything! From your overall look, feel, and health, to your energy levels (both mental and physical), your moods and mood stability, your mental and physical abilities, and even how fast or slowly you age and die (from "natural" causes), you are severely impacted by what you choose to put on, in and around you.

The foods you eat can also affect your professional performance and your sex life. It's true what they say; you are what you eat (and drink). If you are telling yourself you are in "sad" shape physically and energetically, it's likely because you are eating a "SAD" diet—the Standard American Diet, which could more accurately be called the Standard Advanced Western Civilization Diet these days. To perform optimally in all areas of your life, you need to fuel yourself optimally with the right foods, at the right times and for the right reasons. That absolutely does not mean you have to settle for bland, boring, tasteless, and expensive foods. I will get into this a little later in the chapter.

What you choose to fuel your body with directly and impressively affects everything!

We have become so technologically and scientifically advanced that we have forgotten (or chosen to ignore) the core, vital, basic, elemental things about our very own natures—those natures that we have evolved into. The SAD is particularly problematic when it comes to eating to support your basic needs and nature. You eat all the wrong foods, leading to poor overall energy and health. Eating the wrong foods also causes ailments, illnesses, issues, problems, the need to consistently seek out "specialists," pills, potions, or new fads to help you. But, all of those problems could have been prevented if you had just chosen to eat the right foods and make the right choices in the first place. Imagine all the extra time and money you would have if you eliminated all the health issues from your life and you just focused on living the life you love.

When you attempt to thwart your body's natural needs and demands with nutrient-poor foods and drinks, you end up paying the price many, many times over, in many, many different ways. Nowadays most people use synthetic pharmaceuticals to heal illness or provide energy in place of good food. This is creating a huge divide between what our bodies

224

need and what we are giving them. The symptoms of this divide are low energy, depression, lack of motivation professionally and personally, and low self-confidence, along with an endless list of ailments. Before you know it, you are in your doctor's or some "specialist's" office with an unexpected health issue or a brand-new label that adds to your already less-than-healthy lifestyle. Talk about being set up to fail before you start.

> Making wise fueling choices while becoming aware of how those choices affect your body can bring you endless benefits, and a lot more happiness and success in all areas of your life.

Remember, it's not your fault. Our health and food systems have not been created with preventative practices and your best interest in mind. Big business wants you to be fat, sick, and tired because then you will consistently give your hard-earned money to them, in the search for a 'fix' for your many problems. Making wise fueling choices while becoming aware of how those choices affect your body can bring you endless benefits, and a lot more happiness and success in all areas of your life. It will empower you to become far more in control, enhance your self-confidence, and allow you to move away from a place of dependency and confusion.

Let's talk about food intake. The average person consumes more food per day than they need, usually due to stress, not fueling your body in the way it needs, and not living the life you really want. If you restrict your caloric intake, you will lose weight—for a while. However, if you're not happy, not fulfilling your needs, living the life you want, and if you don't get enough of the right kind of calories, your body goes into a protection and conservation mode which makes it store more fat.

Timing and portion control play an important part in fueling your body the right way, and the key is educated SMART choices and moderation. Plan your meals and be aware of how much fuel (food) your body really wants and needs. Don't wait until you start to feel full to stop eating, and have your portions planned. When you finish eating the right amount of the right food, your body is fueled, and you don't need seconds and you won't feel hungry again soon.

> ## When you finish eating the right amount of the right food, your body is fueled, and you don't need seconds and you won't feel hungry again soon.

Just like in your car, if you fill the tank with high-quality fuel, that's all you need to do. You don't need extra fuel, and carrying around an extra can of fuel in the trunk will not enhance the performance of your car; in fact, it adds to its load. If you put water in your gas tank, and the gauge still shows full, the car still might run, depending on how much water or bad gas you put in it, but it won't run very well. You wouldn't want to load the family and your luggage into to head out on a long journey with it. No matter how much you pump in or how many extra gallons you have on hand, if it's the wrong fuel, the results will be less than great. If you are confused about how many calories you need a day or how much of what to eat and when to eat it, check out the recipe and nutrition booklets and guides on my website, where I make it very simple and easy for you.

> ## All processed sugar is sugar, and all of it is harmful for your body and mind.

As I stated earlier in the book, sugar is in almost everything that the average person eats. Sugar is the main ingredient in almost anything and everything pre-made and pre-packaged. Did you know that sugar is in most of the so-called 'healthy' stuff too, like snack bars and cereals, and even salads, vitamins, soups, and yogurt? The fact is, most pre-packaged, pre-made, processed, and fast foods are crammed full of sugar, masked and hidden with one name or another. There are at least 61 different names for sugar listed on food labels. It can be hidden in the ingredients by calling it, for instance, high-fructose corn syrup, which should never be eaten. All processed sugar is sugar, and all of it is harmful for your body and mind. If you want, need, and enjoy sweet stuff, simply change the way you eat it. Use natural, unprocessed, unmodified, and unaltered products that enhance your body and mind rather than harm them.

> The reality is, when you eliminate all these processed foods from your diet, your taste buds become much cleaner, meaning you will start to enjoy the natural flavors of things and you will notice many ailments and cravings will just fade away.

If you are fueling your body with clean, fresh foods, your body will get all the natural sugars it wants and needs. Your body doesn't need all the extra sugars, which are added to make things taste better to those addicted to sugar. The reality is, when you eliminate all these processed foods from your diet, your taste buds become much cleaner, meaning you will start to enjoy the natural flavors of things and you will notice many ailments and cravings will just fade away. My clients often comment on how great their food tastes after they've eliminated sugar and processed foods. They are tasting things they never did before, and loving it, and feeling great.

Have you ever wondered why people say, "Eat your breakfast; it's the most important meal of the day?" Imagine how your body feels after a long night of sleeping, repairing, digesting, and restoring. When you wake up, your fuel tank is empty. It's been 10 or more hours since your last fuel intake (meal). Breakfast is the resource that fuels your body and mind, balances your leptin and blood levels, and ensures you avoid those cravings later in the day so you can hit the road with natural energy and feel great all day.

Simply drinking a cup of coffee and having a slice of toast is not going to set your body and mind up for success. It may stimulate your system into motion, but you would be starting out with your tank on empty, burning through your natural energy stores. You spend the rest of your day trying to fill it up while working, so you are playing catch

Reg's Natural You Tweaks

1. Enhance Your Diet by Adding Minerals. Instead of limiting your intake, expand it. Eat more mineral-rich foods. Eating a primarily whole food and locally-grown and raised diet is vital. Food grown and raised in a natural environment, filled with mineral-rich foods from naturally cared for soil will leave your body satisfied and feeling empowered; no more cravings, feelings of being still hungry, mood swings, weight gain, foggy brain, or allergies to deal with. Shopping at your local farmer's market and growing your own foods are two ways to ensure you are eating mineral-rich foods. And, it's a very empowering way to eliminate all the stress, worry, and frustrations of dealing with the negative effects of poor quality foods.

2. Grow Your Own Food. One of the benefits of growing your own food is that you participate in the opportunity to watch something come to life. You become involved with the enhancement and betterment of your own body and environment while helping to improve the earth. This kind of experience will connect you with nature and bring a new awareness to the relationship you have with the foods you eat while relaxing your mind.

Another benefit is that plants clean your air. We spoke earlier about how toxic the air in your home can be. Growing plants in your home will also detoxify the air. You will notice how different your air smells and feels and how it makes you feel. Growing your own food will save you money and time, and it's a great way to meditate and spend a little "you time" slowing down your brain and just being you for a few minutes.

Also, remember when we were discussing energy and how different energy vibrations and levels impact how you feel and how your body and mind perform. Imagine how powerful, healthy, and happy the energy is in anything and everything that you yourself help, support, love, and cherish. This is a very powerful way to empower your own energy. So, go do it—find your local garden center and buy some seeds or a little plant and enjoy the process. If you have no idea how to grow food, start with one little plant. It all happens naturally, after all.

2. Eat Garden-Fresh Food. Have you ever tasted a fresh fruit or vegetable picked right off a naturally-growing tree or plant? It's so delicious and powerful that your body immediately respond to the vitality of fresh grown foods. Have you ever wondered why most kids don't like the veggies that you buy from the store? It's because the energy is low and effected, and the flavor is pretty much non-existent. Kids are naturally pretty smart when they haven't been fully conditioned with all the stuff we are supposed to believe yet, so sometimes it can be very enlightening to watch and listen to what small children naturally do before they are interfered with.

> Imagine how powerful, healthy, and happy the energy is in anything and everything that you yourself help, support, love, and cherish.

I don't like store bought, chemically enhanced, genetically-modified, gassed-for-transport, and scientifically-altered foods either. I literally cannot put that stuff in my mouth, and when I do, I immediately taste and feel the difference in how my body and mind act and feel. I invite you to buy a store-bought cucumber, head of lettuce, handful of spinach, tomato, apple, peach, pear, watermelon, lemon, fish, or any meat, and then buy the same from a local farmer's market that is lovingly grown chemical-free, or try anything you can find or grow wild yourself. Cut them up and place them in separate bowls, then taste the difference, and feel how each one affects your body and mind. You may notice garden- or farm-fresh plants have an amazing calming and fulfilling effect while they enhance your energy and emotional state. You may have seen the YouTube video about the head of corn left out on a post and nailed beside a naturally grown one. If you haven't, I invite you to look it up.

up all day. Bad choices like this are definitely taking you farther away from the success you want and need. The outcome is sugar cravings, headaches, low energy and decreased productivity at work and home. Your body is not a machine, but in some ways, it's very similar to one. You must fuel it, care for it, and maintain it just as you would your car and your home. If you don't care for your body and mind, they just won't work to the best of their ability for you.

What Is SAD Living?

SAD living is unthinking, compliant living. It's the consequence of adopting the Standard American Diet. It's quite difficult to figure out how Western nations, so innovative and scientifically advanced, evolved SAD living. Our desire for a quick fix and easy-to-prepare foods and products initially stemmed from a desire to make our lives easier. But, it has actually done the exact opposite. Our yearning to save time, save money, lose weight fast, fix (or maintain) a health issue, and make our lives easier, healthier, happier, and freer has become the driving force behind countless ailments, illnesses, and negative issues. We have become unbelievably busy people, and for many it has cost them their health, happiness, relationships, careers, reputation, self-worth, and life.

> Our desire for a quick fix and easy-to-prepare foods and products initially stemmed from a desire to make our lives easier.

Not very long ago, even the most technologically and economically superior Western nation, the United States, was still 40% farming-based. Food was supplied locally, and people ate lots of vegetables, fruit, and locally-grown meat. A bit further back, in the Middle Ages, sugar was sold as a drug in Europe. How times have changed. An instinctive desire for simplicity has created our modern world of damaging and enslaving foods and habits. We now have a false need for inexpensive but fast-energy-inducing foods and products, which have combined with a simultaneous decrease in physical and clear mental activity with an alarming effect.

Over the centuries, our lifestyles have changed dramatically. We don't need to put on the fat we once did. Until a few decades ago, most jobs involved some sort of manual labor. Now, only 2% of the American economy runs on agriculture. Most people work in offices. But, don't be alarmed; our farms are more productive than ever before thanks to technology.

> We have become unbelievably busy people, and for many it has cost them their health, happiness, relationships, careers, reputation, self-worth, and life.

Inexpensive, fast-energy-inducing foods are little more than drugs, as the above sugar anecdote demonstrates. Just think about all of the inexpensive on-the-go snacks available: individually packaged snack cakes, candy bars, and even pre-packaged salads and "healthy" foods that are highly processed and loaded with sugar, or carbohydrates our bodies quickly break down into sugar. These foods lower our energy and vibration levels, and they are the most common and easy-to-buy foods available. You can get this stuff pretty much everywhere and anywhere, and if you can't get to it, there are many ways to have it delivered to you almost instantly. But these days, if you want great, easy, nutritious, natural, great tasting chemical and GMO-free foods that empower and enhance your body and mind, it takes work, effort, research and time. Why do you think that is? The biggest change—and one of the biggest problems—is our busy lives, meaning we don't prepare nutritious meals at home where we are in control of the ingredients and food that we put in our bodies.

The SAD is combined with misguided and misunderstood official dietary advice. The "war on cholesterol" is a good example. It should really be a "war on not getting enough magnesium," since cholesterol is so important to our bodies that when we don't get enough of it from our diet, we make it internally. But, we need magnesium for our bodies to use cholesterol efficiently, and we are sadly deficient in getting this important mineral into our bodies these days.

We spend so much time counting calories, watching our cholesterol intake, and believing that if we eat and drink truly tasteless nutrients, we will somehow lose weight and feel more alive and energized. We get so distracted that we forget the importance of just living, enjoying, experiencing, and learning. Calories don't matter in and of themselves. Starving yourself of cholesterol does not work either. In fact, it is as unhealthy for your body as becoming overweight. Plus, eating tasteless food make most people miserable, increases stress, and causes a person's emotional state to have negative effects on their body, mind, and attitude.

> An instinctive desire for simplicity has created our modern world of damaging and enslaving foods and habits.

To put it simply, if your body, emotions, and energy levels are suffering, you are not living the right way for *you* or making the right choices about the foods and products you surround and fuel yourself with. If you feel tired all the time, if you feel moody or even depressed, or if you just don't feel like yourself, you need to take a good hard look at what you're eating so you can begin to build awareness of how what you're eating is affecting your life.

Cut Out These Foods

So, which foods do you need to cut out of your diet if you want to be healthy, reverse and eliminate ailments and illnesses, lose unwanted pounds, feel better, look better, and gain natural energy? There are probably few surprises in this list, but I promise that you'll feel better when you cut these things out of your diet. After a short time, you won't even miss them!

FRIED FOODS

Vegetable and processed oils are terrible for your body. They are high in trans fats, which throw off the body's much-needed balance of omega-6 and omega-3 fatty acids. Also, once these oils are heated, they can become rancid and are extremely toxic for your system. Processed oils are also one of the major contributing factors to sunburns and sensitive skin, and they greatly contribute to the need for all those sun-blocking chemicals (which are medically proven to be a major contributor to skin cancer) on your body all summer long. If you burn quickly and easily in the summer sun, take a good close look at the foods and products you are putting in and on your body.

The breading that goes along with most deep-fried foods helps your body pack on more unwanted pounds, lowers your energy, and it also raises your risk of getting adult-onset (type 2) diabetes. To make fried foods healthy, you would have to make them at home and be highly selective about the ingredients you used to make them. My suggestion: cut them out altogether and replace deep-fried with my three favorites; barbecuing, grilling, and steaming. Cooking anything from fresh veggies to fish fillets and wild game allows them to cook in their own juices and retain all that natural goodness. Plus, you get to play and experiment with infusing all different types of flavors, spices, and aromas to enhance the energetic and healing properties of your food, along with the flavors and smells. Food and food preparation can be as enjoyable and as empowering as eating the food.

You could also try poaching, broiling, stir-frying, cooking *en papillote*, slow-cooking, pressure-cooking, and even no cooking! There are endless awesome raw food recipes available online. Have some fun, be adventurous with the kids, or try it for a romantic date night. The fun of creating great tasting and fulfilling foods together can be magical and very erotic.

> To put it simply, if your body, emotions, and energy levels are suffering, you are not living the right way for *you* or making the right choices about the foods and products or people you surround and fuel yourself with.

What about microwaves? Well, I'm not going to go into the endless reasons to avoid these horrible machines now, but the fact that they completely destroy any food or liquid you put in them, leaving that food completely useless for your body's needs, should be reason enough. If you own one, stop reading now, go into your kitchen, unplug it and get it out of your house. Replace your microwave with a convection steam oven; it does the job better, healthier, and is just as fast.

FAST FOOD

"Food" you find in fast food restaurants is loaded with unhealthy breads, trans fats, sugars, unpronounceable chemicals, vegetable and corn oils, and a lot of other stuff that would turn you green if you actually checked the ingredients list. Fast food and drinks are also filled with high fructose corn syrup (HFCS). HFCS is very close to the top of the "worst ingredient in the world" list today, and because it's so cheap it's almost ubiquitous. Then, throw in the empty carbs, highly processed ingredients, and refined sugars, and you have the majority of what makes up fast food.

These foods are energetically dead. They are like putting water in the tank of your car. The gauge will show full, but the engine has no use for the stuff. Not only does this stuff not fuel your body, it does exactly the opposite. It lowers your energy and vibration, it negatively affects how your body and mind function, and it makes your body work harder to store what you've consumed and clear it out.

Smart choices are only smart when you have all the facts.

I am not saying this to make you feel guilty about eating fast food, but I believe it's important to know the facts and the significance of these ingredients, which creates awareness, which helps you to understand whether a choice is helping or harming you. Smart choices are only smart when you have all the facts. When you are putting cheap foods loaded with chemicals into your body, you are telling your body it doesn't matter and has no value to you. Is that what you want your body to think or believe? Is that what *you* want to believe about yourself?

BAKED GOODS

Commercial baked goods are terrible for your health. They are loaded with refined sugar and bleached wheat flour, another "empty carb" that's processed like sugar by your body. Commercially-sold baked goods are harmful to your body because the laws of economics mean that manufacturers need to use the cheapest ingredients available. Not only that, but they must load them up with preservatives and fillers so that the food doesn't spoil during shipping, and so it has a sufficiently long shelf life. There are really great baked goods recipes that you can research and make at home, and those recipes are healthier, more fulfilling, and a great way to find more great-tasting foods that not only make you feel great, but look great too.

DIET DESSERTS (MOST NOTORIOUSLY, FROZEN DESSERTS)

Think you're being slick and getting around the health-compromising baked goods with these? You've got another thing coming. Diet desserts substitute artificial sweeteners for sugar and hydrogenated oils (usually soybean oil, one of the worst) or lab-created trans fats for natural fats, so that you still get the taste of an all-natural dessert while having a "healthy" pleasure. Don't be fooled. You're better off eating the sugar- and fat-laden "unhealthy" dessert than these chemically-created concoctions. Diet desserts are nothing less than slow-killing poisons. When you discover the joy and endless benefits learning for yourself, and you get your friends and family involved with making your own foods and treats, you will wonder why you ever ate that energetically-dead, physically- and mentally-destroying stuff at all.

> When you discover the joy and endless benefits learning for yourself, and you get your friends and family involved with making your own foods and treats, you will wonder why you ever ate that energetically-dead, physically- and mentally-destroying stuff at all.

SODA POP

I'm sure you've seen the YouTube videos showing all the things people can do with these "refreshing" sodas. If you can strip 30 years of rust off your cars bumper with this stuff, why would you ever pour it into your body?

Whether it's called "soda" or "pop," it's always slow death in a bottle if you drink too much of it. Who doesn't love an ice-cold pop, or some other soda product every now and then? But, if your main beverage of choice is soda, you're just killing yourself with an overflow of sugar and synthetic chemicals. Worse yet, food and beverage companies typically use HFCS in place of sugar, making it five times worse for your health. A major cola company just admitted that they have understated the health risks of their products, and its direct link to many of the top illnesses around today. If a company has finally been forced to admit it "may cause some harm," you can imagine how bad this stuff really is. Many of these drinks have been directly linked to cancer due to the ingredients that are responsible for making the drink you love so much taste the way it does.

If you think you're skirting this matter by drinking diet soda, you're in for a big shock. Diet soda is probably the worst beverage that you can put into your body, short of a certified liquid poison. It's a chemical factory, and its artificial sweeteners are directly proven to cause cancer, neurological damage, and other harms to your body. Diet soda is a prime example of how we have drifted away from acknowledging the needs and demands that our bodies are asking for. Don't believe me? Do a little research on your own. If you don't care and you think I'm just wanting to make your life difficult by scaring you away from all the stuff you love, then you are reading the wrong book!

What is the Best Fuel for Your Body and Mind?

Simply put, the best fuel for your body and mind is alive, fresh, and natural. By this alive, I mean food that is now or was recently living. It is food you don't need to check the label on, you don't need to count the calories with, and you don't have to wonder when, where and how it was made, and what kind of energy was put into it, or how much of it you should or could eat. It's simply real food in its natural form— plants (fruits and vegetables), nuts and seeds, fish, poultry, and natural whole grains grown from Mother Earth's seeds and soil, with nothing added or taken away. These foods are rich in inflammation-fighting antioxidants and phytochemicals. They help the body produce and activate enzymes that are necessary for hormone production and chemical reactions in the body. In addition to these foods, foods rich in probiotics and prebiotics are also considered "alive," as they help promote the healthy bacteria in your body that are the first line of your immune system.

So, what exactly is "dead" food? If it can sit on your counter for days or weeks and not go bad, then it's a dead food. These foods are refined, highly processed, often synthetic, and have little or no nutritional value. Think about foods like cheese-flavored crackers, meal replacement bars, fruit snacks, and flavored beverages. They all include some sort of manmade chemicals, artificial colors, and flavors. If the stuff you're putting in your body is filled with ingredients on the label that you can't pronounce, then it is "dead" food.

I make every option available to spend time with and learn from the wise and experienced.

Get to know your local fresh food suppliers and avoid the center aisles of the grocery store. You are a unique individual with your own weight and bone structure. You have your own metabolic body type (ectomorph, endomorph, or mesomorph). You have your own tastes in foods and drinks. You have your own medical history based on lifestyle and genetics. You have your own goals and your own dreams about what you want to achieve in terms of career, personal fulfillment, and longevity. And, you have your own way of choosing to use your body and take care of it. Stop filling your only body with a bunch of stuff produced by people you don't know and enjoy the power of making your own food choices to empower your body and mind.

I make every option available to spend time with and learn from the wise and experienced. One hobby I have is making friends with people who have been there and done that. I invite them to get involved with my projects and hobbies. This is a huge win/win situation for endless reasons. If you wish to learn how to eat naturally, empowering your mind and health, ask an old farmer (or the wife of the farmer) to give you some cooking lessons. You will bring a lot of happiness and value to them, and the lessons you will learn are priceless.

Yes, there are basic, elemental things that you should be fueling your body with to meet your body's needs, and yes, you do need to live in harmony on this planet, so being rigid is not a harmonious way to live. Yes, our bodies are incredible, and yes, our bodies can deal with living on a full diet of processed and dead foods. The goal is not to stress yourself out and live in a bubble, but to educate yourself, become aware of how you feel, what affects you, and what empowers you. If you love chocolate cake and a bottle of wine, have it, enjoy it, savor it, and love it, but be very aware of your goals and dreams so that you can use foods like this to empower you rather then stifle you. As you gain knowledge and experience, you can refine what you do, when you do, and how much of it you can do, then add or subtract from there.

What are the basic ways of fueling the body for optimal health? Here are some general guidelines:

Eat healthy fats and proteins. Vegans have a hard time with this. The mass media promote veganism because it's fashionable, but long-term, and depending on their blood type, vegans often have many issues that are generally not seen as connected.

Eat low-sugar and low-carb foods. If you need to lose a bit of body fat, you should cut way down on your natural sugars and carbs intake, but never cut them out entirely. As a 'normal' person, living a 'normal' lifestyle, your body does not need a lot of natural sugars or carbs, but they are needed. Professional athletes are an important exception to this rule. They need to be on high-intake of a very well-balanced diet, especially a day or two before a competition. Carbs provide the fuel your body needs, so don't ever cut them out completely. Just moderate how much and how often you eat them, depending on your lifestyle. When you do eat carbs, make sure they're coming from a high-quality, whole-food source. I have a chart on my website you can download for free.

Add in omega fatty acids. Omega fatty acids are healthy fats that are essential to many processes in the body. Plus, getting in enough omega-3s can help protect your heart, and protect your body from cancer, too. Be mindful of getting omega fatty acids in 2:1 or 3:1 proportions. My favorite is Udo's 3-6-9 blend; I take it every day.

Eat your veggies. Eat fresh vegetables with every meal; even eating a small portion regularly will make your body very happy. Again, get adventurous and experiment with all the great colors and flavors available. Do your best to eat in season and support your local organic farmer. There are so many different types of veggies, and endless ways to prepare them, or you can just eat them raw. If you or your kids don't like veggies, learn to prepare them in different ways. The internet is crammed full with endless ways to use veggies, so have fun with it.

Eat the right kind of meat. If you eat animal protein, such as red meat and seafood, do your best to find a local hunter or supplier to buy from. You should eat organic, wild, fresh meat if you're going to eat it. There are a number of websites online where you can order direct and get fresh, natural foods delivered right to your home or office. Eat more light meats then red. With all your meats, but especially red meat, be sure to buy wild or grass-fed beef, beefalo, bison, deer, elk, caribou, moose or other game to ensure it is toxin-free—and to be sure the animals are more humanely treated during their lifetimes. Following this rule means the energy you put in you is that of something healthy and vibrant, rather then something scared, abused, and drugged up.

We spend so much time counting calories, watching our cholesterol intake, and believing that if we eat and drink truly tasteless nutrients, we will somehow lose weight and feel more alive and energized.

Remember, we can control this planet, and the way things are done, by voting with our money. If the thought of an animal living its entire life in a dirty, dark cage, being shot full of chemicals every day bothers you, then stop buying meat from the grocery stores. If everyone would just stop supporting these big businesses, they would have to change the way they do business. Ignoring it all, and blindly handing over your cash to companies strategically working to make you sick will not make things better, and the government and the FDA are doing nothing to help you. If we don't all choose to force a change for our own good and the good of our future families, who will?

Reg's Natural You Tweaks

1. Eliminate Typical Snack Foods. Depending on the goals of your health and fitness program, there's nothing wrong with snacking from time to time. But, the foods that have somehow become the traditional snack foods in Western society are SAD indeed. Again, we find bucket-loads of bleached wheat flour, refined sugars, empty carbs and starch, vegetable oils, and nutritionally-worthless table salt. Note that sea salt not only tastes better, but it is also nutritionally richer. Except on very special occasions, you're going to have to militantly avoid pretzels, potato chips, baked crackers of all kinds, and similar foods if you want to have optimal health. Or, you could simply choose to make your own.

2. Avoid Breakfast Cereal. The breakfast cereal business may seem innocent, yet it is one of the most harmful industries in our world today. Even cereals that are considered "good" encourage excessive grain-eating, which has been found to *not* be good for the human body. Science now tells us that eating an abundance of modern-day grains leads to health problems. Why? Because we are not eating the same stuff our parents or grandparents use to eat. Big business has us by the throat. Everything has been changed, refined, locked, and protected. You can't patent nature, so they are eliminating nature to scientifically create stuff that they can patent, which is pretty much everything on the shelves today. Plus, these cereals are loaded with sugar and all kinds of other fillers, stabilizers, enhancers, and preservatives, too. Most people then add commercially-sold, nutritionally-worthless pasteurized milk, which causes lactic acid build-up that leads to muscle cramping and the build-up of phlegm. No wonder everyone is allergic to everything these days. A great book on this topic I suggest you read is *The China Study* by T. Colin Campbell and Thomas M. Campbell.

3. Make Your Own Energy bars. Most energy bars are just expensive candy. They are loaded with substances that break down into sugars in the body, and they're loaded with quick-energy-fix substances, too. You may as well save your money and eat a Snickers bar in most cases, although there are notable exceptions. If you make your own, you can control the ingredients and ensure you are getting the whole food health benefits energy bars are supposed to provide.

4. Eat More Greens. If you have ever had a plain lettuce salad (especially iceberg lettuce) from your local restaurant and wondered why you don't like salads, it's because they are plain nasty, boring plate of lettuce. They are not salads. These unexciting 'healthy food offerings' are usually made with some chemically-enhanced and gassed GMO version of something green. Would you like a sandwich that was only made up of nothing but bread? Would you even call it a sandwich? What about a sandwich with just bread and one other ingredient? Still boring!

5. Get adventurous. Try replacing your usual lunchtime sandwiches with a big salad made with mixed leafy greens of all different flavors and colors, a wonderful variety of colorful veggies and seasoned with fresh herbs and natural oils, and possibly topped with organic chicken, tuna, or wild turkey. Use your imagination. Put a bunch of different types of lettuce in there, chop up some cucumber, kale, okra, scallions, celery, onion, peppers, radishes, shallots, beans, tomatoes, broccoli, cauliflower, a few pieces of fresh apple, pear, blueberries, acai berries, bilberries, strawberries, blackberries, cherries, or plums. Then, sprinkle a few mixed nuts and seeds over it, like flaxseeds, pumpkin seeds, sunflower seeds, sacha inchi seeds, and chia seeds. Try adding some lemongrass, fresh mint, or something completely different. I love to mix all kinds of combinations that can be made into salads, soups, stews, breads, deserts, protein shakes, snacks, and full meals. Squeeze a lemon, lime, apple, orange, or other fruit all over it all with a light drizzle of organic, cold-pressed hemp oil, coconut oil, avocado oil, or extra virgin olive oil—or all of them. Yummy! Try eating a bowl full of this at lunchtime and see how your body and mind performs for the afternoon, Then, see how well you sleep that night.

Eat berries. Berries may be the most nutritious of the fruit-foods, and they make a great dessert as well as a great snack. There are so many things you can do with berries, and so many things you can add them to. There are endless recipes and ideas online. Start experimenting and enjoy the endless possibilities.

Eat nuts and seeds. Nuts and seeds (such as roasted sunflower seeds, pumpkin seeds, almonds, hemp seeds, and the such) are some of the best sources of non-animal healthy fats and proteins. Plus, they're loaded with many micro-nutrients that are not only essential for your body to function properly, but they can help prevent diseases like cancer, too. Nuts and seeds make a great easy alternative dessert or snack, and they will fill you up faster. They will also give your body and mind the natural energy you need to keep going through the day, without an energy crash or mood swings. They are easy to pack, light to carry, and taste great both on their own and mixed with other fruits and berries. You can eat them raw, cook them, and make endless snacks with them. On the weekends I mix up a big batch of different concoctions, individually package them up, and freeze them. I have food for months that easily fits in my pocket, bag, suitcase, glove box in my car, gym bag, briefcase, desk drawer, and pretty much anywhere else I need them to be. There are so many of them, I never get bored with them or the combination of things I can make with them. They're a win-win snack.

Here is a list of the nuts and seeds I like:

Nuts:

Almond	Chinese Almond	English Walnuts
Australian Nut	Chinese Chestnut	Filbert
Beech	Chinkapin	Florida Almond
Black Walnut	Chufa Nut	*Gevuina avellana*
Blanched Almond	Cobnut	Gingko Nut
Brazil Nut	Colocynth	Hazelnut
Butternut	Country Walnut	Heartnut
Candle Nut	Cream Nut	Hickory Nut
Candlenut	*Cucurbita ficifolia*	Horned Water
Cashew	Earth Almond	Chestnut
Chestnuts	Earth Nut	Indian Beech

Indian Nut	Para Nut	Rush Nut
Japanese Walnut	Paradise Nut	Sapucaya Nut
Java Almond	Pecan	Sapucia Nut
Jesuit Nut	Persian Walnuts	Shagbark Hickory
Juniper Berry	Pili Nut	Sliced Almonds
Kluwak Nuts	Pine Nut	Slivered Almond
Kola Nut	Pine Nut	Sweet Almond
Macadamia	Pinyon	Sweet Chestnut
Malabar Chestnut	Pistachio Nut	*Terminalia* Catappa
Mamoncillo	Pistacia	Tiger Nut
Maya Nut	Polynesian	Walnut
Mongongo	Chestnut	Water Caltrop
Oak Acorns	Queensland Nut	White Nut
Ogbono Nut	Royal Walnuts	White Walnut

Seeds:

Chia seeds	Poppy seed	Safflower
Flaxseed	Pumpkin seeds	Sunflower
Hemp seeds	Sesame seed	

Learn how to cook with plantains. Plantains in some parts of the world are called "dinner bananas." They are a delicious superfood.

Learn how to cook with herbs and spices. When you think of "spicy" food, do you think "hot" or "full of flavor"? For me, spices are all about the flavor and enhancing the flavor of the foods I'm making. When you flavor the natural foods you eat with natural herbs and spices, you don't need huge amounts of table salt, refined sugar, or a bunch of chemically-enhanced sauces and condiments all over it, to make a healthy meal taste delicious. Fresh herbs and spices have many, many possibilities to enhance and empower your food, which will enhance and empower your body and mind. They also have a lot of their own health benefits too. For example, many are absolutely loaded with healthy antioxidants. I have a great little booklet about herbs available on my website.

Drink non-dairy milk. Drink non-dairy milk. Drink pure and natural almond milk, hemp milk, spelt milk, oat milk, hazelnut milk, coconut milk or rice milk. You can make these at home very easily. These drinks are filled with nutrients, taste great, and are healthy and delicious natural foods to enhance endless meals and snacks. Try them on your home-made granola cereal, in your organic coffee, or in your home-made smoothies. Make your own ice cream, tasty treats, deserts, and snacks. You can even make your own butter, yogurt, and more. *Try them*—they taste far better than you may imagine and your body will love it.

Make healthier sweet baked goods at home. Substitute your old processed, dead flour for pure hemp protein powder, and use a natural sweetener like honey, cane sugar, or maple syrup rather than sugars or artificial sweeteners. Find a local bee farmer and buy your honey from them. It supports your local community, and it gives your body all the tasty, sweet joy it wants and needs while empowering your immune system. Or, if you have space, invite your own family of bees into your yard and make your own honey. The new beehives are awesome and easy to use. No smoke or no special suits; just you and the bees living harmoniously and supporting each other. How empowering is that?!

If you live in a city area, drink water filtered by reverse osmosis. As we covered previously in the book, put getting high-quality filtered water at the top of your priority list. Adding filtered water to your home is one of the best choices you can make to live a happy, healthy, and successful life. Too many people have forgotten the pure, refreshing joy of drinking pure, clean water.

Replace your soda. And, replace any other high-caffeine, high-sugar (or HFCS/chemical sweetener) beverages with water, herbal tea sweetened with honey, or lemonade using pure lemon juice. Make your own fresh juices, too: try adding a bit of fruit into your vegetable juices, or add a little bit of vegetable into your fruit juices. Have fun with it—*try it*! They satisfy your thirst more than sugary drinks and they fuel your body too, leading to better health and longer lasting, natural energy.

Eat hemp-based products. The proteins in hemp-based products are a great substitute for protein powders, especially dairy-based protein powders, which I strongly recommend you avoid totally. Pure organic

Reg's Natural You Tweaks

Drink Ionized Water: Drinking water has a massive impact on your overall health. Get into the habit—do it all day, every day, and the results will be more amazing than you could ever imagine. The vital key to drinking water is to invest in a high-quality reverse osmosis unit and a water ionizer to ensure you are drinking pure, clean water. Most unfiltered drinking water and bottled water is full of stuff your body doesn't need. That water also has traces of toxins like fluoride, and it is stripped of essential minerals vital for good health. Ionized water is super powerful. It can degrease your oven and clean your BBQ. Imagine how much money you would save—not to mention the health benefits you'd get—from drinking it. Using a high-quality reverse osmosis unit and water ionizer provides your body with the ultimate natural cleanser. Drinking ionized alkaline water will gradually lower the body's acidity and enable the body to dispose of its waste products. An alkaline system can live longer and function better.

hemp products now abound, and you will be amazed at how good they are and what they will do for your health and your energy levels!

Remember, whatever you do, avoid HFCS as if it's the plague (it is), and avoid "white bread" products and most other "white" foods, as they are basically devoid of nutrients. Don't believe me? Try a white bread meal for lunch and see if you want to fall asleep at your desk afterward. Instead, try an exciting, flavorful, and colorful high-protein salad, like I mentioned earlier. Or, try one made with sliced boiled eggs, an apple, and an orange squeezed then shredded. Add couple of chopped dates, a handful of mixed seeds and nuts, sliced organic chicken, turkey, tuna, wild steak, sardines, or anchovies, and some organic avocado and coconut oil poured over it. You'll feel alert all afternoon. Mmm, I'm going to go make one now!

Detoxing

One of the most important aspects of fueling the body (and that I touched on briefly earlier in the book) is detoxing the body of the unnecessary toxins our bodies have built up. Releasing toxins allows the body to be replenished with the nutrients and minerals it needs to thrive.

We are surrounded by synthetic chemicals in our everyday lives, and our bodies absorb those chemicals. When we use plastic bottles and bags, detergents, synthetic soaps, shampoos, and household cleaners—not to mention pharmaceuticals—we are putting unmeasurable amounts of toxins into our bodies every day and lowering our natural vibration and energy. Optimal performance becomes challenging, and it affects how successful and happy we feel in our lives.

> One of the most natural ways we detox the body is by drinking pure, clean water.

The body's immune system is so powerful that we don't even notice these toxins. But, over the course of many years their effects build up, so that one day 'all of a sudden' we mysteriously find ourselves ill, run down, or just not as healthy as we intuitively know we should be.

There's more. As I already mentioned, our foods are often laden with toxins these days. For instance, we buy beef that comes from factory-farmed cattle that are chemically-boosted and genetically-altered, corn-fed animals, and are thus very unhealthy, with very low and negative energy. These cows are regularly shot full of antibiotics to keep them alive and in decent health while they are crammed into dark, dingy barns. They're also pumped full of hormones to make them grow bigger. Do you realize that when you eat any food, whether it's meat, fruit, or veggies, that is pumped full of all these chemicals, it may be possible that these chemicals may also get absorbed by you? Every time you buy that fast food burger, buy low-quality foods, or even red meat from a higher-end restaurant, you are consuming the same stuff these things grew in or were fed.

> Your body is not a machine, but in some ways, it's very similar to one.

The same goes for fish. We buy fish because it's healthy, but we forget about the possibility of heavy metal poisoning (especially from mercury), a risk especially high when eating predatory fish like tuna. Farmed fish usually aren't any better; they're often raised in cramped tanks full of dirty water.

Worse yet, many of the toxins in our foods these days aren't even recognized as such. For instance, you have already read about HFCS, which is as toxic as it gets. But, you've likely been gobbling it down because it's everywhere. Only very mindful eating and paying careful attention to food and beverage labels gives you the possibility of avoiding it.

So how do you start detoxing your body to remove the chemicals you've been accumulating for decades? One of the most natural ways we detox the body is by drinking pure, clean water. I'm not taking about that stuff stored in plastic bottles and sitting around for many months on a dock somewhere. It's recommended to drink 3–4 quarts or liters of purified water a day because this naturally cleanses the body. If your urine is yellow, or even dark or brownish and smelly, you definitely need to drink more water.

Several other ways of detoxing include taking natural detox dietary supplements, going to an infrared sauna for 30 minutes a few times per month, taking a salt bath regularly, sitting in a sweat-lodge, and exercising. I'd like to draw your attention to a couple of other methods that I highly recommend to the people I work with:

- **21-day water fasting.** I know it sounds crazy, but I do this every year. Try it before you judge it. It will change everything. It is vital before starting any fasting program that you follow the prep and break instructions prior to starting. This detox needs to be approached with caution, using mineral water or filter-purified water only. I do this twice a year, in the spring and the fall. You can also do mini-water fasts, such as a 24 hour fast, weekend fast, seven-day fast, and so on. Visit my website for more information on water fasting. I will give you tips and provide support to help you achieve new levels of mental clarity, energy, and vitality.

- **A temporary (several day) juicing and raw-food diet.** This is another great detox to do several times a year. You will be amazed at how great you feel after a 7-day pure juice fast.

There are many other detoxing programs to consider, including:

- Blood cleansing
- Parasite cleansing
- Lymphatic drainage
- Colon flush
- Liver flush
- Kidney flush

You can research these various methods in greater detail to get a better idea of what is best for your unique body and physiology, but always remember to educate yourself. Remember what I said early on in the book regarding detoxing. Be aware, make smart choices, and learn how your body naturally functions, and use what you learn to follow the natural route to the best way to detox your body. Detoxing should be done periodically, but not constantly. Depending on your lifestyle and they type of detox you wish to use, once every two months works great for many people who are in relatively good health, if not most people. I suggest doing complete systems cleanse at least once per year, and doing mini-sessions all year round. If you're suffering from or dealing with ailments, issues and chronic problems, contact me. I'll help you step into and through the right program for you.

Make Sleep a Priority

Fueling your body with the right stuff to be the best, natural version of yourself goes beyond what you put in your mouth. You have to fuel your body with rest, too. Sleeping between 11 p.m. and 5 a.m. is vital to help your mind, body, and organs repair and maintain themselves. People who claim they can do just fine on four hours of sleep a night or less are only fooling themselves and setting themselves up for disease, injury, and eventually, a long vacation in the local hospital—or worse.

Endless studies prove that lack of sleep causes issues such as slow mental and memory function, weight gain, muscle fatigue, low libido, sexual dysfunction, decreased sex drive, slower reflexes, concentration problems, mood swings, depression, high blood pressure, diabetes, low immunity, disease, and countless other negative effects. Yet, many of us still aren't making sleep a priority. If you want to be the best version of yourself, you must get better sleep, and more of it.

Inadequate sleep interferes with the body's ability to metabolize carbohydrates and causes high blood levels of glucose, increased insulin levels, and greater body fat storage. Low-quality sleep and irregular eating habits drive down leptin levels, increases cravings for simple carbohydrates, and reduces levels of growth hormone—a protein that helps regulate the body's proportions of fat and muscle. This can lead to insulin resistance, contribute to an increased risk of diabetes, and increase blood pressure and risk of heart disease.

Let's consider the story of a boxer who has a dream to be a world champion. He is in the ring everyday training. He eats all the right food and gets to bed early every night because he knows how important sleep is for his body to recover. He eats, sleeps, and focuses on his goal and everything he can do to achieve it. The day comes to get in the ring, the bell rings and WHAM! With one punch he knocks out his opponent and becomes the world champion.

Now what? Suddenly he has managers and sponsors pulling him all over the place for TV, radio, and magazine interviews. He is invited to all the best parties and his life becomes a buffet of endless options. (Sounds like my kind of party.) With his new lifestyle as world champion and an endless list of opponents ready to fight, how will he maintain what he has?

The boxer lived a clean, healthy lifestyle, with the dream of getting to the top of his game. But once he won the championship, it completely changed the amount of sleep he was getting. He was so busy partying that he never got any sleep, and he suffered for it. Getting less sleep greatly affected his ability to maintain his high level of mental and physical performance. The same is true for you, whether you're trying to get into the C-suite, or you're wanting to be the best parent you can be. Sleep needs to be at the top of your 'must-do' list and scheduled into your daily calendar.

High-quality sleep requires a good quality bed (remember how important your environment is!) and commitment to a schedule that prioritizes at least eight hours of sleep per night. Pay attention to how your body feels when you get up in the morning. If you notice aches and pains right away, you may need to invest in a better-quality bed.

If you are not getting enough sleep, keep track of what you are doing before bed. Ask yourself:

- What are you eating and drinking?
- Where are your electronics?
- What's the air quality like where you sleep?

- What kind of lighting do you have?
- Whom are you sleeping with?
- What's going on in your mind?

For the next three days, be very aware of your sleep and see if you are creating a schedule and an environment that will support you to get plenty of quality sleep.

What can you do if you don't like what you find? Turning off all electronics at least an hour or two before sleeping will really increase the quality of your sleep. Spend your last hours awake by candlelight and completely away from all electronics. Try actually talking with the people you share your space with, or read a great book. Relax, unwind, and shut off. Make sure your bedroom is dark, with no light source at all in your room. Pick out your favorite essential oil and fill up your aromatherapy diffuser. And, make sure your big green leafy plants are happy, well fed, watered, and are happy in their little environments. You may be quite surprised at how much better you sleep.

Create "Super-Cells" to Fuel Your Body

Your body is, of course, made up of cells. The healthier your body's cells are, the more efficiently your immune system and other systems can work. In other words, "an ounce of prevention is worth a pound of cure."

How can you create and maintain super-cells in your body? There are many easy ways to do this:

- **Eat whole natural foods and drink pure clean water.** Drink beverages without added sugar and artificial flavors.

- **Avoid processed, pre-made and fast foods.**

- **Stay physically active.**

- **Get plenty of high-quality sleep.**

- **Keep your hands clean.** It's shocking that even many doctors don't wash their hands as often as they should. Your hands are constantly around your mouth, having already touched everything around your house or office. If they aren't clean, you aren't clean, and your immune system will be over-wrought with attempts to cleanse you. Avoid the antibacterial soaps, go natural, or even better, make your own and add a few drops of pure essential oil into it for a great smell and natural way to kill off bacterial visitors, without killing off your immune system.

- **Keep the mold and mildew out of your home.** Shampoo your furniture and rugs a few times per year with natural cleaners or steam alone. You can do this yourself or hire the pros to come in; either way, insist on chemical-free, natural cleaning. Have your heating vents cleaned out semi-annually. Keep your bathroom, refrigerator/freezer units, and bedding clean. If you can afford a very high-powered vacuum cleaner that works highly efficiently whether the bag is full or not and one that is customized to clean windows and doors, buy it.

- **Be safe with your sex life.** It's frightening how many serious infections and diseases can be engendered by sexual activity. Even just kissing and body contact can share infections and more. Be smart in your choice of bedmates, and whomever you share your energy with or give it to. There is no truth in "meaningless sex." Everyone you share your time and energy with either gives to you or takes from you. Use protection, and don't hesitate to see your doctor at the slightest sign of a possible STD.

- **Learn how to breathe better.** Shallow breathing is habitual today but deep breathing is one of the best, easiest, and least expensive ways of cleansing the body. Oxygen is a key factor to removing illness and disease from your body and having a strong immune system. So, learn to breathe using the full capacity of your lungs, and ensure the air you are breathing in is fresh and clean. Get into and enjoy nature, near seawater and trees, as often as possible.

Are you filling your gas tank with regular gas, unleaded gas, premium-grade fuel, or a mixture of some great fuel with a bit of dirty water?

You can't expect to look like a million bucks when you eat from the dollar menu! A healthy, natural life will not only help you sleep better and reduce your pain, but it will also improve your energy levels and sex life, making life better for you overall. What you fuel your body with is tremendously important, so pay attention to what you eat. The relationship you have with food will play a key role in the food choices you make for yourself. Again, I can't stress enough how powerful you are. Your body is your mechanism to create and maintain high levels of natural energy, health, happiness, and success. Are you filling your gas tank with regular gas, unleaded gas, premium-grade fuel, or a mixture of some great fuel with a bit of dirty water?

Key Takeaways:

Everyone has a different relationship with food, and no one diet will ever work for everyone. Everyone's nutritional needs are unique. Developing a healthy relationship with food is what optimal nutrition is about.

Choose foods and ways of cooking that ignite your passion, empower and fuel your lifestyle, and make you jump out of bed with excitement in the morning.

You must fuel your body, care for it, and maintain it just as you would your car and its fuel and oil tanks. Don't skip breakfast, and make sure you eat a lot of great-tasting, natural, whole, fresh foods and liquids.

Reject SAD living—the so-called 'normal' living that comes with consuming the Standard American Diet.

Smart, systematic detoxing regularly gives your body the opportunity to replenish its cells with the nutrients and minerals it needs to reach optimal performance.

Filtered, cleaned and ionized water naturally cleanses your body and your home.

maintaining your Results

"

Mentorship is an
incredibly huge
responsibility. And you
need to choose your
mentors carefully, just
like mentors choose
their apprentices
carefully. There has
to be trust there, on a
very deep level.

— JIMMY CHIN

Support Systems and Coaching

Throughout this book I have provided small lifestyle tweaks you can easily make to bring you closer to being a more natural you. This book was inspired by my frustration with how our Western culture, systems, and mindsets have created a world where people are fat, sick, confused, frustrated, stressed out, and unhappy. I believe in a world where we all are inspired and connected to one another. In this new world, people are in alignment with what brings them fulfillment, happiness, health, and success, and they support each other to get there and stay there. Of course, a successful, happy, and healthy life looks different for everyone, but wouldn't it be great to know that the communities you are part of are filled with people who are committed to being the best versions of themselves? You see, it's in empowering and supportive communities that people can achieve and maintain positive and successful changes in their lives long-term, while at the same time helping others to do the same.

> This book was inspired by my frustration with how our Western culture, systems, and mindsets have created a world where people are fat, sick, confused, frustrated, stressed out, and unhappy.

Have you ever tried to give up something because you know it's not good for you, but the people and environments you live and work around are filled with encouragement to keep doing that thing rather than stopping? You can abstain for a while, but eventually the temptation becomes too much. You find yourself adding that thing back into your life. You may feel guilt and shame or feel discouraged about your lack of will power. Guess what? It's not your fault. No one would be able to maintain their results in those kinds of conditions. That is why it's so important to develop a system of support when you are making changes for your life.

> It's not your fault. No one would be able to maintain their results in those kinds of conditions.

In the last chapter of this book I want to share different ways you can create a support system for yourself and your life. I wondered for years why people would keep coming back to me and other practitioners with the same ailments and complaints—then it hit me. People need community, mentors, and coaches. We all need people who care, really listen, truly want to see you succeed, and are willing to support you in doing so. Your support system can be the difference between achieving what you truly want or failing. Set yourself up for success, because ultimately, it's your life! This is not a dress rehearsal and no one is going to change your life for you. This is it. This is your time to take control and become the empowered and magnificent version of the natural you. It's your long-term health, happiness, and success that are at stake.

Everybody Needs a Support System

How many times have you embarked on a journey to transform something in your life, made some progress, but then ended up right back where you started? Maybe it was something as challenging as giving up a specific food, cigarettes, or drinking. Maybe you were dieting and managed to lose 25 pounds. You were doing well, and you were making progress on the 20 more you had to lose. Then suddenly, you put on 10 again. What happened? You didn't have the right support system.

Support systems are key to breaking habits that aren't serving your greatest self, and they are extremely important to maintaining those changes, too. If you don't have the support you need to create and maintain change in your life, you will go back to your bad habits and bad choices. If you're not constantly working to move up the hill toward your wants and needs, you'll slide back down.

What do support systems look like in your life?

Support can look like a blog you follow, a group you are in where others are committed to achieving similar goals, or encouraging family members, friends, and/or work colleagues. The coaching industry is booming right now because people need support and mentoring from others who are traveling on similar (yet unique) journeys to become better versions of themselves, both professionally and personally. And, because everything is connected, how you are showing up for yourself in your personal relationships is how you are showing up in your professional ones too. Remember what we said about this in previous chapters. Be smart when it comes to choosing your coach, mentor and support groups.

If you've ever had the disheartening experience I described above— of successfully accomplishing a goal that really empowered your life, and then feeling stuck again a few months later—it's probably because you lacked support, or worse, possibly because you surrounded yourself with old friends or the usual gang of people who have no desire to change, and they don't want you to change either.

Sometimes you need support from people who don't know you to really reach outside your old life and become consistently committed to living a life that you love. An outsider can give you the tough love that the people closest to you often don't or can't. Working with the right person one-on-one can help you create that experience. If you want to truly make a permanent change in your life, the key is to ensure your environment and the people in it are supporting your new journey. And, you must choose to work with someone one-on-one who will be a part of it all while you're on the journey.

I am committed to supporting you in being the best version of you. The Natural You approach I have created and outlined in this book will give you a foundation. To help give you even more support, I'm building a community right now that's also available to you through my Ultimate Health University at www.reglenney.com.

If you are looking to work consistently on your goals of achieving and maintaining an extraordinary and powerful life, this is the place you want to be. It's a community of people who want to support one another in attaining their goals professionally and personally. In this community, the students are all using the Natural You approach, just like you. It's a group of people who want the same thing you want—to live an extraordinary life—and who are all using the same framework to get there.

As a member of my community, you will receive support from me through group programs and online classes, which you can do at your own pace. Plus, you will be the first to be invited to participate at live, in-person events, retreats, and courses all around the world. As a member of our support group, you will also have preferred access and special discounted pricing to extra support from me directly. You can ask your questions, voice your concerns, discuss your frustrations and fears. I will even work with you to help create your very own personalized programs to ensure you are on the right path to your long-term health, happiness, and success, using the same techniques I've used with celebrities, members of royal families, and other highly successful people around the world.

It's All About You—But You Can't Do It Alone!

One of the most powerful things that highly successful people do is to ask for help. More than that, they know that asking for help is only the first step. What is truly vital to their long-term success is to accept the help and choose every day to implement the smart choices needed to ensure they achieve, maintain, and enjoy the time, effort, and money invested. At some point, you need to stop going from one illness to another, one "specialist" to another, one diet to another, one training program to another, one relationship to another, and one stressful life to another. And, you need to stop giving the best of you to your job or to others.

The world's most successful people may give a lot to others, but this usually originates from a passion and drive to continually improve *themselves* in all areas of their lives. To do this, they need to achieve a balance that enables them to enjoy their success and grow it. And, they don't attempt it alone. After a while, most successful people find that they need a place to go where they can recharge, where they can discover how to stay on top of their game, and how to maintain a high level of mental and physical performance.

> At some point, you need to stop going from one illness to another, one "specialist" to another, one diet to another, one training program to another, one relationship to another, and one stressful life to another.

When changes come thick and fast in life, it's difficult to maintain your focus on the things that matter most and to achieve a balance. But, just because it's difficult doesn't mean that it's impossible. You must learn the techniques and strategies to get there, swallow your ego and pride, and accept and implement the right strategies. Then, you can enjoy the incredible success that those steps bring you long term.

What Can a Gifted Life Coach Do for You?

A gifted life coach is one who has many years of real-life experience, one who has personally gone through the fire, and one who has a natural ability and desire to consistently improve him- or herself while maintaining a passion for his or her work and the success of others. Natural gifts and talent are far more powerful then educated knowledge, but when you bring the two together, exceptional things can happen.

A naturally-gifted, highly-educated coach, one who has a lifetime of real-life experience, will treat you as a unique and holistic being who requires unique and individualized guidance and support. They will take all aspects of you and your life into consideration and ensure you are able to implement the right steps at the right time into all aspects of your life. A gifted coach will take you beyond another high-energy self-help event that's just more information to put on your shelf. They will be your guide and support to finally achieve what you always knew you could.

A gifted coach will take all aspects of you and your life into consideration. This means that your life coach will get to know every aspect of who you are and how you function to ensure you can achieve and maintain high levels of mental and physical performance while enjoying ongoing change and success daily. They will also have the life experiences and professional training required to support you through all your growth and challenges. In short, they will have all of the tried and tested strategies and techniques needed to support you holistically in your exciting journey through the changes you need to implement into your daily life so that your life fulfills your wants and needs long term.

A professional coach adopts a highly personalized and tailored approach based on your unique needs and goals. He or she will have a finely-crafted system full of the strategies and techniques used by the other successful people they have helped. The right coach will use this experience to design the ultimate lifestyle coaching program that will work specifically for you. A true professional life coach will be there for you when you need it; you won't be scheduled into an hour slot a couple times a week or month, regardless of when you need help. High-level success comes from support when you need it and keeping you on the right path, no matter what.

The result:

- You will enjoy regular growth, change, improvement, enhancement, and success.

- You will discover and maintain higher levels of happiness, health, energy, creativity, productivity, motivation, and fulfillment.

- You will feel invigorated, but also have a sense of calm and clarity as you are stimulated to achieve your purposes and set new, perhaps more ambitious, goals for your future.

- You will begin to live as you have never lived before, enjoying happier and more fulfilling 'you' time with far less stress.

For you to achieve and maintain exceptional results while implementing the various steps described in this book in an organized and coordinated way, it makes sense to work with a coach who has been there, done that, and who is passionate about helping you create your own exceptional life, too.

> In short, they will have all of the tried and tested strategies and techniques needed to support you holistically in your exciting journey through the changes you need to implement into your daily life so that your life fulfills your wants and needs long term.

The perfect coach will help you bring together all of the disparate parts of your life to work in harmony so that you achieve the joyful relationships, professional success, abundant health, and fulfillment of dreams that you want and need to achieve, resulting in a better, more fulfilled you.

The Right Coach for You

There is no shortage of "certified coaches" in the world today. There are even more selling themselves as a "professional Coach", who have no professional training at all. Often times, these are just people who have gone through difficult experiences and then saw an ad encouraging them to "be a coach" or "write your book." These "specialists" may have taken a short course, usually online, and are now out there and excited to work with you. There are even many online coaches who are just really great sales people, full of excitement and promises, but not able to offer any real substance. Their website is awesome, they say all the right things and promise you the world, yet when you get into their courses and guidance, you quickly see that it is a lot more like the average fad diet or celebrity fitness program: it's a one-size-fits-all program where everyone is told to do the same thing, or you're told what you need to do without any guidance and support to step you though exactly HOW to do it.

> There are many online coaches who are just really great sales people.

People are increasingly turning away from traditional psychiatrists, and for good reason. But, it's even worse to put your life, your mind, and your future into the hands of a passionate individual who has little or no real training or life experience in all the areas you need to get clarity in, and focus on, if you're going to be successful in all areas of your life. Just like a fad detox program that's designed to work on just one aspect of your body without taking all the others into consideration, working like this often times doesn't work long term. And, even more worrying, it can be detrimental to all the other areas of your life.

Be very careful of the marketing scams. In this day and age we are bombarded with "Specialists" and "Professionals". Almost everyone these days is one. Social media is full of individuals making bold statements, claiming their beliefs as fact, when the real facts are quite different. I see this every day on social media, someone posts information regarding a health issue, then hundreds of individuals spew their beliefs as fact, with no real knowledge or facts about the topic. Everyone has an opinion and they often get very aggressive about it. This is why there is so much confusion about it all. Even more worrying, many times individuals take the on-line advice as fact, incorporate it into their lives and end up with very bad experiences. Then you read that "alternative therapies don't work". Well, of course they don't work when they are done wrong or being directed by someone who has no real clue about what they are talking about. The worst thing you can do is ask for advice about anything on social media.

> If you are going to put your life and your future into the hands of someone else, anyone else, whether it be a doctor or a coach, you must take an honest look at that individual, ask a lot of questions, find out about their life, and take a real hard look at how they look, act and feel.

What about the marketing on-line where you yourself can become a "professional" anything, just by paying a bit of money and taking a few hours worth of training, to learn to say the right things and "build your own successful business"?

There are countless websites and great online marketing where you can hire a 'professional coach', as well as learn how to become a

"Professional Coach" yourself, within just a few days. Really! There is one organization in particular claiming to hold the "Gold standard in coaching", yet in as little as 2.5 days, they will give you the very powerful title of "Certified Coach", allowing you to go out in the world and help others. Personally, I have been dealing with countless organizations and individuals who are "highly trained professionals", claiming to train, support and hold to "higher standards" their 'professional coaches'. One organization in particular claims to "leads the industry with its own Code of Ethics", however the facts are quite different. I have personally witnessed the life altering damage these 'professional coaches' can cause. When a complaint was issued via their "complaint department" clearly outlining the damage these coaches have done, along with proof of dramatically un-ethical behavior in their personal and professional life, the association was not even interested in discussing it. The real goal of these associations is money, and keeping as many paying members as possible.

Organizations making such powerful statements such as; "taken the lead in developing a definition and philosophy of coaching and establishing ethical standards among its members." And claiming they have created the "gold standard in the coaching world" are dangerous! Many organizations like this who make statements, such as; "What the world needs right now is a few more coaches", need to come with a large warning disclaimer. What they really are saying is "we want more people to join our association and pay us a monthly fee". The reality is, these companies are profit driven, not high quality. Their interest should be put into the right kind of high quality training along with monitoring and demanding that the coaches who represent this powerful and life altering profession are the most highly qualified and professionally trained individuals possible, showing it and living it in their own personal and professional life.

A "professional Coach" must be held to a higher standard and they must live that in every aspect of their lives, so as to help others by their own actions and the highly trained services they provide. These organizations are pumping out coaches as fast as they can, in fact, you can become a professional accredited coach in just 60 hours! That's only 2.5 days! If you really want to reach the top of their "professional coach association", then all you need to do is pay them money and dedicate a maximum of 2500 hours, or an easy 3 - 6 months, and this is their best-trained coach. How can anyone with only 3-6 months worth of online or classroom training, working with a few of their friends and family as test subjects, be a highly trained coach that represent a "Master Certified Coach" title? This is not only very bad for the coaching industry, this is very, very bad for those individuals giving their hard earned money and trusting their lives to anyone with this title. It is belittling and damaging our entire profession. It is one thing to be trained to say all the right words to come across like a professional who can truly support an individual going through tough times or wishing to 'get to the next level", it is entirely a different thing to actually have the skills to do it right.

> The list of circumstances and situations that a life coach can help you with goes on and on, but a true professional will remove the pressure from you and guide you through the journey with as little pressure and time possible, while you enjoy the new energy, empowerment, and growth.

Be very, very careful when searching for a "highly trained specialist", so you do not end up trusting your life and your future to anyone who is simply after your money while doing their best to help you. Just because an organization has a lot of members and located globally, does not guarantee the coach you give your hard earned money to and trust your life and future to has the complete skills, personality, ethics and higher standard to guide you through all that is required to create the life you want and need.

Do your research, be very clear about who you invite into your life and into your head, and make sure the "professional" has far more then a measly 2.5 days – 6 months worth of basic training before given the title of "professional Coach", "certified Coach" or "Master Certified Coach".

How to Make a Choice

How often do we feel fully alive and make choices that are true to who we are?

Life can be challenging, and we can get stuck in ways of being that are judgmental, doubtful, bitter, and worrying, to name a few. Life can also be exciting, exhilarating, and inspiring. The power to change your life is in your beliefs, and beliefs play a huge role in the choices you will make in your everyday life.

| I hear it all the time: "laser focus!"

You can have limiting beliefs that hold you down and back, or you can believe that change, growth, and success can happen for you effortlessly.

Its time to make a stand! Be an adult! Find the way!

I have spent over 32 years working with people you could consider highly successful—actors, singers, professional athletes, business owners, corporate leaders, politicians, and royal families. When working with me and my programs, the biggest turning point in the journey is when clients start paying attention to the choices they were making due to their beliefs, and why they were making those choices. Some make choices in reaction to their environment, some make choices because they are afraid of an outcome, and some make choices because it's what they strongly believe in. I have had conversations with people in their 80's and 90's still making life choices based on the fear their parents instilled into them, even when they know it is wrong, or doing things they would rather not be doing. The key is to know if those choices are benefiting you long term. Are the choices you are making keeping you accountable to your success, or are they taking away from it?

Choice even comes into play when finding and creating your support systems. I began to successfully maintain my success as soon I discovered how important it was to invest in having a mentor in my life. Before that, I was a lone ranger. I could do anything I put my mind to, but *man*, was that a lonely road. Opening up to the idea of investing in myself by getting someone to support me in achieving new levels of success was life-changing.

THIS IS HOW I UNDERSTAND MENTORSHIP:

M OTIVATES YOU to accomplish more than you think you can.

E XPECTS the best of you.

N EVER GIVES UP on you or lets you give up on yourself.

T ELLS YOU THE TRUTH, even when it hurts.

O CCASIONALLY kicks your butt.

R EALLY CARES about you and your success and invests as much time in you as needed.

Choosing to invest in yourself isn't always an easy choice. Some see it as selfish, and that belief becomes a block to achieving higher levels of happiness, success, and health. Not only that, but you might worry about what other people think of you. Some may think you are self-centered. Some may judge you for it. Some may even say, "You are already successful, aren't you happy with what you have?" Or the big one: "How could you afford that?" But what kinds of people are making those type of statements? Are these people highly successful? Are they regularly achieving great success in all areas of their lives? Do these people want you to be happy, healthy, and highly successful?

Unfortunately, most people let this kind of feedback or negative thinking stop them from living an extraordinary life that creates a level of happiness, success, and health they could only dream of.

The point I am making here is that when it comes to upgrading your success, happiness, and health, you are going to have a moment where you will get to choose what it's worth to you. What are you worth, and what is your life or business worth?

What is more expensive—working toward your goals on your own, working to overcome your bad habits and find motivation on your own, or working with a mentor who has done it and been there, a mentor who knows the hurdles and challenges and has the strategies and techniques to successfully bring you through them? How have your choices worked out for you so far? Where are you right now, even after all the 'trying'? How much more time and money will you spend on 'trying' more? How many more relationships will you go through, how much more weight will you gain, how much more money will you lose, or how sick will you get before you choose that enough is enough?

This is what it looks like when you go it alone: you spend time and money going from one strategy to another, one office to another, from one program to another, trying to take what you learn and implement it into your own life, in your own way. You don't really feel the way you want to feel, and you don't really achieve your goals—and even if you do achieve them, you don't maintain what you worked so hard for. More often than not, you're losing everything you worked so hard for. Often times while focusing so hard on the challenge right in front of you, you're missing all the small details on the sides, not to mention letting your health, your family, and your 'You' slip away.

> How many more relationships will you go through, how much more weight will you gain, how much more money will you lose, or how sick will you get before you choose that enough is enough?

What could you achieve rapidly if you worked with a mentor or coach one-on-one, who customized the right program for you? You would get a mentor who empowers you and stands for you and your success. You would have your very own supporter to encourage you when you wanted to give up.

What could you achieve with a coach who even has the option for you to join a community of people to support you? You could be seen and heard if you chose, and you would get feedback from others if you wanted or needed it. You would inspire others with your magnificence. And, you would maintain your results with ease because you had the support you needed, when you needed it. You would have a community of people on a similar mission, standing with you shoulder-to-shoulder, achieving goals and turning dreams into reality. With these types of powerful and inspirational people on your side, your only limits are the ones you put on yourself. And imagine the awesome business opportunities, too!

What are the choices you are making right now that are supporting your happiness, success, and health? Do you have a community to support you? Do you have a mentor who can pick you up when you fall? Do you have a mentor who will keep pushing you forward, even when it feels uncomfortable?

The choices you make are always yours, and they will always be based on what you believe. Remember, too, your environments play such a huge role in your beliefs. Please use the 10 Keys to Ultimate Happiness, Success, and Health and notice how they all work together. You will find that you begin to see amazing results in your life. Visit reglenney.com and you will see the results I have supported people in achieving. I love the work I do, and I would love it if you chose to join us in empowering ourselves while we help to empower others. I guarantee you will quickly experience exciting changes and growth. If you don't, I'll give you your money back.

My motivation is to support people to not be sick, stuck, and tired anymore. My mission is to support already successful people in the world to take their personal and professional lives to a place that fulfills, empowers, and encourages them, and makes them feel really happy. I want to show you how you can maintain that level of greatness and achieve more. A lot of successful people plateau and think they have reached a ceiling in their success. I say that if you have already hit your ceiling and done all you can do, then the really exciting stuff is just a couple of easy steps away. Let's acknowledge the amazing success you've already achieved and see what else you can do for yourself, your family, and your community.

Key Takeaways

Support systems are key to breaking habits that aren't serving your greatest self, and they are extremely important to maintain those changes too.

It's also key to work with a naturally-gifted, highly-educated and seasoned coach or mentor one-on-one, someone who has your best interest in mind, and who has the strategies, techniques, and community for you to be a part of while on the journey.

You could try to excel with the help of family members, friends, work colleagues, online blogs, or the endless "specialists" available to you. Or, you could choose to get support from someone who has all the tools, strategies, and techniques in place to ensure you stop 'trying' and start achieving now. How will you get the support you need to make the changes you want and need in your life?

A talented and committed life coach will treat you as a unique and holistic being, looking at all aspects of your life, including your beliefs, environment, relationships, fears, what's holing you back, and what makes you excel. A talented coach will guide and support you through tiny, easy-to-implement, easy-to-maintain steps every day. Those steps will produce the biggest positive changes to help you become the ultimate natural version of you.

Before committing to a coach, do your research!

"

We all have the
extraordinary coded
within us, waiting
to be released.

—JEAN HOUSTON

conclusion

Everything you experience in life affects how your body and mind work. Your body is a powerful healer, and the wisdom you naturally have can support you to create a life you love. The relationships you have with food, people, and the places you live and work in can provide you with the information you need to be the best natural version of you, or you can allow them to slowly kill you.

Conventional medicine, cultural impairments, and the systematic dysfunction I've discussed in this book are not supporting you to be naturally you. Big business and the world we now live in are designed to keep you down, confused, frustrated, sick, and broke. Now you have the information you need to begin making a different impact on the community you live in by committing to making small tweaks here and there that will support natural changes in your life.

As you research yourself, you begin to learn what it means to *be you*. You discover what you need and what works best for you and your health, happiness, and success. This guide is here to reference any time you are feeling stuck in your life or struggling with dis-ease in your body or mind. The great thing about the Natural You approach is that you can tune in at any time, take responsibility for your life, and create extraordinary results that you will be able to maintain.

Hopefully by now you are convinced that you don't need to be the tired, grouchy grizzly bear.

It really doesn't matter if you are 18 to 39, 40 to 59, or 60 or above. Regardless of your age, you can have a better body, better health, a better quality of life—and a better you. There is no point in living a life of endless suffering, sickness, and deterioration. If you have turned into a grizzly bear, reverse it, and become your invigorated self again. If you haven't yet become a grizzly bear, then prevent it from happening.

Your quality of life is in your hands.

Your choices are empowered by your knowledge and your beliefs. Make the time, get clear about your beliefs, be honest with yourself, and do all you can to ensure that your choices become your power, rather then your pain.

The Ultimate Health University

If you want to take yourself and your physique to the next level, don't skip the next few pages.

My holistic approach to health and lifestyle has been helping people live in stronger, healthier, better bodies since 1988. Those who take action, incorporate what they have learned, make a stand, and find the way to follow what I teach will enjoy great results. I personally guarantee it. However, those who take the *next* step and get personalized coaching and lifestyle coaching with my customized programs—well, they're the people getting *extraordinary* results!

> Conventional medicine, cultural impairments, and the systematic dysfunction I've discussed in this book are not supporting you to be naturally you.

This may all seem easy, and it can be. You keep hearing that losing weight is harder than it sounds, but at the Ultimate Health University, we have a healthy lifestyle and weight-loss program that is designed to teach you how to lose weight and keep it off, while at the same time improving all aspects of your life, enabling you to become a happier, healthier, more successful version of you. We will give you the knowledge, support, and tools necessary to lose weight and become healthy long term.

So why do participants achieve extraordinary results? Not only do they receive the very best "innovative" information and training, but they know that there is a helping hand to support them along the way, day in and day out. They know that one-on-one support is crucial to their success, and that they cannot achieve the extraordinary success without it. As the saying goes, "no one succeeds alone." If you research anyone who is at the top of their game—whether it's in sports, singing, the corporate world, entrepreneurship, or any other high-level industry— all the top performers have worked with mentors and coaches to get there, and they still work with mentors and coaches to keep them there.

We have many different programs available online at ultimatehealthuniversity.com.

You can join us at one of our events, workshops, or retreats. My team and I can create a customized corporate program for your office or team, or I can work with you in person and customize exactly what you need and want.

Make no mistake—my Ultimate Health Transformation Program is not your average health program. It's based on over 32 years of tried, tested, and proven real-life strategies that really work. After experiencing this fabulous program, your health and fitness will be taken to an entirely different level of dynamic power and success, not just for the weekend, but for the rest of your life.

Take the first step to becoming a better, natural you and sign up today.

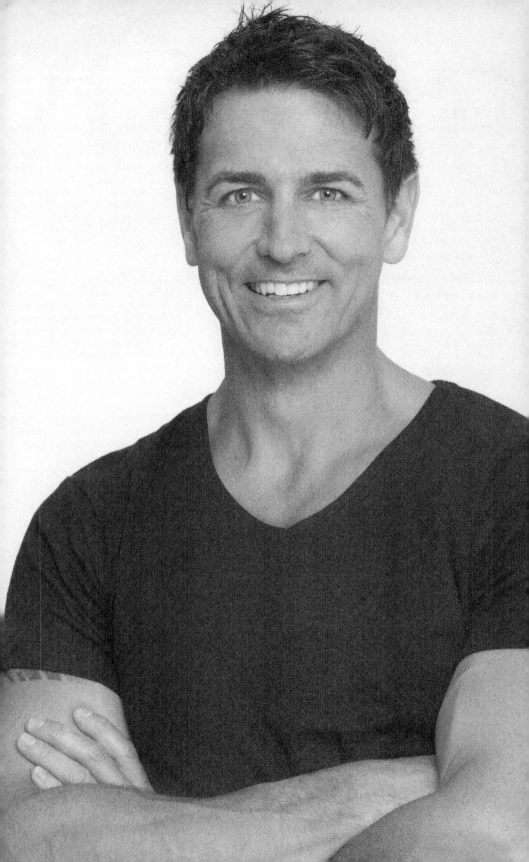

About the Author

Reg Lenney, The Multi Award Winning Vital Coach, known as 'The Ultimate Natural Health Coach,' is an executive lifestyle coach who is highly regarded and called upon by many professional athletes, Fortune 500 CEOs, singers, bands, multiple royal families, and Hollywood A-list celebrities such as Wesley Snipes, Susan Sarandon, Pierce Bronson, Patrick Stewart, Mel Harris, Mario Bello, Kevin Bacon, Halle Berry, Britney Spears, Al Pacino, and Courtney Love, to name but a few.

His programs are based on achieving and maintaining exceptionally high levels of mental and physical performance and enhanced lifestyle. He is known for guiding his clients to eliminate chronic aches, pains, ailments, and disease while helping them understand the effects your beliefs have on your lifestyle, choices, habits, relationships, and environment, and how all of those elements combined ensure you live the life you love, or take you away from it. Now renowned as The Executive Lifestyle Coach to the stars, Reg is responsible for creating some of the most famous physiques in fashion, music, politics, and industry. He helps you to systematically detox and cleanse your body, and fuel your body in the right way for your body and needs. And, he helps you create a fitness program that works in the right ways for your body, fits into your lifestyle, and achieves your goals. He can help you to eliminate pain through muscle balancing, energy balancing, and body alignment to create a powerful and balanced, pain- and ailment-free, healthy body and mind.

Along with numerous articles, magazines and TV shows that Reg has been featured in, he is also regularly commissioned to work with many top companies and both private and public individuals wishing to achieve top performance and results. Reg has a passion for getting to the core of a problem so as to "fix" issues and take his clients to new levels of health and performance in all aspects of their lives. Everything you do affects how your body and mind works. Reg's passion is in guiding his clients through the strategies and techniques he has developed over 32 years of training and real-life face-to-face experience with people of all levels from around the world. Following Reg's easy-to-implement strategies will ensure you have the power and knowledge to take control of your health and life so you can live the life you love and love the life you live.

Printed in Great Britain
by Amazon